Food, Teens & Behavior

BARBARA REED, PhD

with

Scott Knickelbine &

Mark Knickelbine

FOOD, TEENS AND BEHAVIOR
A Natural Press Paperback

Printed in the United States of America

Natural Press
A Division of Natural Enterprises
P.O. Box 2107
Manitowoc, WI 54220

Library of Congress
Catalog Card Number 82-063-208

ISBN 0-939956-04-7

Distributed by Contemporary Books, Chicago, IL

This book is dedicated to my son, Trace, and his wife Lauren, and to my husband, Paul.

ACKNOWLEDGEMENTS

A first book is always something of a milestone, and so I'd like to take this opportunity to thank not only those who made this volume possible, but also all the people who have influenced and helped me along the way:

My appreciation, first, to Dr. Gayelord Hauser, for his book *Look Younger and Live Longer*. Hauser's book triggered my own awareness of the connection between diet, health and behavior — and saved my life as well.

I am grateful to Judges Frank Bayer, James M. Bierce and William B. Pike of the Municipal Court of Cuyahoga Falls, Ohio, for their cooperation and support as I developed my nutritional program for probationers.

I must thank Alice Kalita and the Huxley Institute for Biosocial Research for their work in informing the public about the links between diet and crime.

Special thanks must go to Timothy D. Schellhardt of the *Wall Street Journal,* whose front-page article on my work gave rise to a spot on the CBS Weekend News, the chance to testify before Senator McGovern's Select Committee on Nutrition and Human Needs, and from there to media appearances and speaking engagements all over the country. This exposure has encouraged other probation departments, correctional institutions and programs for the behaviorally-impaired to experiment with the orthomolecular approach.

I owe an inestimable debt of gratitude to Dr. John Baron of Cleveland, Ohio and biochemist Oscar Rasmussen, Ph.D., for their patient and consistent help with many of my probationers whose lives were in shambles, and who are now living examples of what biochemical correction can do. My thanks also to Carl, for patiently accepting the long hours of work and travel necessary for me to develop the program.

My appreciation to my assistant at the Municipal Court of Cuyahoga Falls, Betty Criss, for her years of loyal and conscientious help with the direction of the many lives our probation department touched.

The staff at Natural Press are to be commended for their

work in completing a project of this size. Special thanks to Scott Knickelbine, who directed research and writing, Debra Lovelien for her cover design and production management, and the tireless Ellen Bonnin for her input at every stage of the book. Thanks to Betty Durbin and T. Walz, who proofread manuscript and galley.

A number of very distinguished professionals took time to read earlier drafts of the manuscript, and to make valuable suggestions. Among these I must thank Linus Pauling, Abram Hoffer, Bernard Rimland, Marshall Mandel, Carl Reich, William Crook, Lendon Smith, Thomas Hartmann, and Michael B. Schachter, all of whom have built towering reputations in the field of orthomolecular medicine and research. Thanks as well to nutritionist Ruth Yale Long, Ph.D., Judge Robert J. Moore, psychotherapist Mary L. Friedel, psychiatrist Elezar Kadile, and criminal justice officials Robert E. Golden, Ted Hanchett, F.R. Marburger and Daniel MacDougald.

To all these, and to hundreds of others, my heartfelt thanks. What gratitude I have earned by popularizing the link between Food, Teens and Behavior must be shared by you all.

Barbara J. Reed
Manitowoc, Wisconsin
December 16, 1982

TABLE OF CONTENTS

FOREWORD

Barbara Reed and I have arrived at our conclusions about the biochemical connection between diet and noncompliant behavior through different routes. She got the message from her own biochemistry; she knew she wasn't crazy (she's not) but why did her brain fog up one day? She also had enough sense to realize that others might be trying to operate using a brain on "tilt."

My path to the truth that biochemical abnormalities will alter behavior was via the confusion surrounding the cause and treatment of hyperactivity. I realized that not all hyper kids had been brain damaged during birth or the neonatal period. I began to ask about hereditary factors. I found that 60 percent of the members of families containing hyperactive children had diabetes, obesity, or alcoholism — all sugar based problems. I decided to ask a question, "What do you eat for breakfast?"

Barbara was doing the same thing 2,000 miles away. We were finding a universal truism. If the neocortex of the brain is not nourished optimally, the conscience, the humaneness and perceptions of reality are not operative or are distorted.

We all have a "selfish, mean and I'll-get-what-I-want" department ready to take over when the "nice" brain is not functioning.

Research indicates that 75 percent of prisoners were hyperactive as kids. So the children I am trying to help are the same ones Barbara may get later on. I have the feeling that if we don't help these children when they are children their parents, the school, and their peers will put them down and they will get the *bad self-image,* the sine qua non of crime.

Barbara's followup indicates that these probationers will not go back to crime if they stick to the program. I like that. I want the program to work.

We have waited too long for other theories — bad seed, social problems, psychogenic factors — to be tested and found wanting.

Her book and the cleverly intertwined case histories with research findings of all the bright people in the health field are very persuasive. No more testing or studies are necessary; we must simply implement the diet in pregnancy as a preventive; in infancy, childhood, and adolescence as a control for hyperactivity, allergies and infections in adulthood before they slip into crime. Most of these children I see because of school failure simply do not feel good. This is exactly what Barbara is telling us. We must be better skilled at reading the bodies of these children. One question gives them away: "Is he a Jekyll and Hyde?"

There is no psychiatric condition that makes a person such a changeling. These mood swings are a result of the victim operating under the control of different layers of the brain — sometimes the human brain, sometimes the animal brain. I can't count the number of times a mother has told me, "He had murder in his eyes!" And the child was only three years old!

Keep the neocortex fed and the rest of the body will conform. The brain and the body **are** connected.

This book should be required reading for all parents, criminologists, psychiatrists, social workers, police people, judges, wardens, or anyone who takes care of other people.

Can we get state legislatures to vote a three-bean salad, whole wheat bread, fresh fruit and nuts as snacks for their state prisoners? Barbara and I would guarantee fewer riots.

Lendon H. Smith, M.D.

CHAPTER ONE
ENLIGHTENMENT

"Enlighten the people generally, and tyranny and oppressions of body and mind will vanish like evil at the dawn of day."

— Thomas Jefferson

This case was different. As chief probation officer for the Cuyahoga Falls Municipal Court, I usually handled misdemeanor offenses — nothing more serious than shoplifting or disorderly conduct. I wasn't used to this kind of crime.

Murder, after all, is the ultimate crime.

I got a call from one of our police officers that morning. "Barbara," he said, "I think we have a case for you. Kid tried to kill his girlfriend last night. He missed, luckily, but he ended up shooting her in the hand. He seems like a bright young guy, but he's pretty messed up. Maybe you can do something with him."

The officer filled me in on the hard facts: At 11:40 the previous evening, a

23-year-old man, whom I'll call Raymond, had been arrested for wounding his girlfriend with a Smith and Wesson .357 Magnum. Apparently he had tried to shoot her in the head; at the last second she deflected the gun, and the bullet went through her left hand. In the light of day, both Raymond and his live-in girlfriend insisted that the shooting was an accident, so the most that Raymond could be charged with was "discharging a firearm within the city limits."

But we knew the shooting was no accident. In the first place, a .357 Magnum is the second deadliest — and the second heaviest — handgun in existence. One does not lift the heavy Pistol and trip the cumbersome firing mechanism by accident. Secondly, Raymond was no stranger to firearms. He had been a champion marksman for several years, and was qualified to handle any type of pistol with the utmost accuracy. There could be no doubt — this was a clear case of attempted murder. And had Raymond succeeded, there might have been a grisly aftermath: there was another bullet in the gun, possibly for himself.

The police records reveal only confusing glimpses of what happened that night. This is Raymond's disoriented account:

> After I came home from work and we had supper, Ruth (not her real name) said she wanted to go visit an old friend and I was going out to a friend's house so she told me where she was going and I told her where I was going...I felt that our relationship wasn't what I thought it was and decided I was going to leave for a-while...Just then Ruth came home and saw I was leaving. We sat down to talk for a few minutes and I wanted to leave. I got up to go and she wanted me to stay. I said no I want you to stay here, and we were struggling and the gun went off only 5-10 seconds later. My friend came in and helped us to the hospital.

But the picture Raymond's girlfriend gave us was quite different. She revealed that the friend she went to visit was actually an old boyfriend, and that Raymond had called his place several times that night. They didn't answer the phone, so Raymond thought the worst.

When Ruth arrived home, Raymond's bizarre behavior began, she said. He began by pulling her jeans down around her ankles and loudly accusing her of making love to her ex-boyfriend. After some verbal abuse, Raymond left the room and retrieved his pistol, loaded with two rounds of ammunition. As he headed out the kitchen door, Ruth thought he intended to kill himself. She ran out to the yard to try to dissuade him; they fought, and Raymond pointed the barrel of the big gun at Ruth's head. He pulled the trigger. She deflected the barrel at the last moment, but the bullet tore a one-inch hole in her left hand. Doctors predicted the hand would be permanently crippled.

Despite his attempt on her life, Ruth refused to believe the man she loved wanted to kill her. She didn't want to see him go to jail, and she was resisting her parents' attempts to get a settlement from Raymond. "I know this was an accident, and I know Raymond loves me, because he does nice things for me and spoils me," she said in her statement to the police.

Of course, Raymond's parents were even more upset at the incident. For them, it was yet another new low in the decline of their son's mental and physical health, a decline they had been helplessly witnessing for nearly 20 years.

Raymond was a bright, vivacious baby, and his parents had high hopes for him. He seemed interested in everything, and it seemed he went directly from crawling to running.

About age four, however, Raymond's parents noticed he suffered from sudden spells of weakness. At times he would tire out so quickly that he had to take food along when he went out to play, in case he needed a sudden pick-up. In grade school, Raymond was a creative child, but his grades were mediocre. He needed special help learning to read, and his mother recalls he seemed to "tune things out."

It was in his early teens, however, that Raymond's behavior became truly disturbing. From around age 13 he began to experience radical mood swings. His grades in high school dropped to C's and D's. He started dating girls a lot in his senior year, and was away from home most of the time. His eating habits — which were never very good — got even worse. His moodiness and depression increased, and in the last half of his final year in high school his grades were abysmal.

After graduation Raymond met Ruth, and eventually the two moved into an apartment together. Although Raymond's physical and emotional decline ceased briefly when he adopted the strict diet required for his competitive shooting, he soon returned to a steady consumption of fast food and snacks. His mood swings were almost manic-depressive: vivacious and self-confident one minute, bitter and depressed the next. Raymond had attempted to kill himself three times before he was arrested. Now that their son had hit rock-bottom, his agonized parents could only wonder, "What went wrong?"

When Raymond was brought to my office the following afternoon, he had just finished making a preliminary court appearance after spending the night in jail. That would be enough to rough up anybody's looks, but I could tell something else was the matter with Raymond. Though polite and cooperative, he seemed detatched, as if he had awakened in a strange and shadowy world. He sat bolt upright in his chair, his hands stiffly locked in his lap, his brown eyes and haggard face displaying little emotion save for an anxiety to which he seemed to have grown oddly accustomed. During the course of our first interview, he even called his girlfriend at the hospital, warmly assuring her he would visit as soon as he could. But I could see Raymond was showing an empty, hackneyed paternalism with no real affection behind it. Somehow I sensed that I had to reach Raymond, and reach him now. I felt that, in a very real way, the rest of his life was hinging on this three-hour interview.

If Raymond had ended up in any of the vast majority of probation offices in this nation, or if he had been one of the thousands of adolescents and other young people sent to correctional institutions or mental hospitals because of chronic behavior problems, he might have been referred to a psychiatrist. The psychiatrist, with the aid of ink blots and pointed questions, would have attempted to discover the developmental deficiencies in Raymond's mind which led to his antisocial behavior, and would have suggested some treatment — probably rap sessions or drugs.

Or perhaps Raymond would have been placed on the rolls of a social worker, one paid by the county or state to help him improve his social lot. Maybe Raymond would have spent several years in prison. If he had received this typical treatment, Raymond would most likely have become one of the seven out of every ten probationers who end up in court again, usually charged with a more serious crime.

I didn't treat Raymond that way. I asked him what he ate.

In fact, I asked him a number of questions about his general health, and discovered that he was a physical and emotional wreck. Raymond suffered from mental confusion, uncontrollable emotions, abdominal pain and a variety of other symptoms — to say nothing of the suicidal tendencies which had led to the incident for which he had been arrested. But I discovered that he was killing himself in a more gradual manner: he ate nothing but processed junk foods. He and his girlfriend were living on donuts and pastry, cheap white bread and pasta, processed canned goods, candy and gallons of coffee. Raymond and Ruth had, in fact, been eating junk a short while before the shooting occurred.

I didn't tinker with Raymond's mind

or try to change his social situation. Instead, I and the doctors at the Baron Clinic in Cleveland modified his diet. As a result, far from being another dismal statistic, Raymond is today a healthy, productive member of society, as are over 80 percent of the probationers who have appeared before me in the ten years since I started my dietary therapy program.

At this point you may be asking yourself. "Where did this Barbara Reed learn to be so successful, if most probation programs throughout the country are so terribly ineffective?" The answer may surprise you: I didn't learn it anywhere from anyone. The fact is that if I had not myself experienced the same kinds of physical and psychological problems which beset my probationers, and learned on my own how to overcome them, most of the more than 5,000 men and women who have had their lives transformed by our program would likely have wound up where they were headed when I first met them — in a hospital, in prison, or dead.

A lucky coincidence? Therein lies the paradox. In the sixties, when I was learning my profession, no one ever mentioned the idea that diet could have any bearing whatsoever on delinquent or antisocial behavior, except perhaps in instances of extreme starvation. We were told that every behavior had its roots in the social history of the subject. Likewise, psychiatrists learned that the cause lay in developmental deficiencies, and doctors were taught either to ignore such problems or prescribe a tranquilizer.

Yet the arrival of the late sixties and seventies heralded the birth of a tiny group of doctors, psychiatrists and others dealing with behavior problems who proposed a link between America's ubiquitous diet of processed foods and the enormous increases in crime, schizophrenia, hyperactivity, learning disabilities and a range of other emotional disorders which had hitherto been assumed to exist in the mysterious realm of the mind. Many of us labored in isolation, never realizing that there were others out there who had made the same discoveries and were having the same successes. In almost every instance these professionals, despite a dismaying lack of academic or clinical research into human nutrition, achieved their enlightenment from personal experience. By solving their own diet-related problems and those of their patients, they saw the obvious link between the way a human body is nourished and the way it behaves.

This may at first sound disheartening; if even doctors have a hard time finding this information, how are lay people supposed to find out about it? Though the question may appear overwhelming, it is in reality a source of great hope.

This book is not written primarily for professionals, but for the millions of parents who fear that they are losing control of their children and who don't know which way to turn. A distorted personality and a criminal record need not be the unavoidable legacy of growing up in the last years of the twentieth century. You don't need a library of child-care books or a live-in psychiatrist to avoid these problems, either. Just as personal experience has enlightened a growing body of professionals, your own personal experience can show you the devastating effects of the typical American diet, as well as the enormous benefits of the proper diet.

Let me tell you my story.

In 1963, the same year in which I became a probation officer in Akron, Ohio, I became seriously ill. My illness was the sort of thing doctors have trouble diagnosing. I developed extreme fatigue and lethargy, and regardless of whether I slept or how much sleep I got, I woke up feeling dead tired. I experienced violent mood changes, going from giddy heights to bleak lows.

Sleeplessness wasn't my only nocturnal problem. I had horrifying nightmares, and would bolt from my bed in a cold sweat. My physical health was also deteriorating. I contracted streptococcus infections in my throat three times in 1963 and 1964.

But perhaps the most frightening symptoms were the memory lapses. I forgot the names of friends, and locations of familiar buildings, and words I had just read. In Akron, my office was located on the ninth floor of the city building and the criminal court was right next door, on the second floor of the old police station. One morning, as was my routine, I left the city building, descended to an underground corridor which joined the buildings, crossed to the police station, performed some minor tasks at the criminal court, returned and took the elevator to my office. What made this morning so unusual was that I was halfway up the elevator, in the midst of a conversation with an attorney, before I realized I had even left my office in the first place! I had carried out my tasks in a complete trance; I could not remember what I had just done, nor even what I had been saying to my lawyer friend, although I saw by the look on his face that I had not been completely incoherent. It was a total blackout. I knew nothing except that I was in one place one moment and in another the next.

This kind of experience scared me into seeking a doctor's advice. My general practitioner gave me the usual examination.

"What is it you do again, Barbara?" he asked.

"I'm a probation officer."

"Oh yes. . .and you have that little boy to take care of, too. I think your problems stem from the stress of working too hard. I'm going to prescribe a tranquilizer."

I didn't want a tranquilizer. If I had problems, I wanted to work them out, not cover them up. I ignored the prescription, but the symptoms I suffered got worse. I sought a second opinion, and the second opinion was more tranquilizers.

I was at a loss, so I decided to play it the doctor's way. But one experience with phenobarbitol was enough for me;

the dizziness, lethargy and confusion I felt seemed worse to me than the original symptoms. I flushed the remainder of the pills down the commode.

In desperation I even asked my gynecologist during the course of a routine exam what he thought the problem might be. His face turned grim. "Barbara," he said, "I'm afraid you're going through the beginning stages of menopause." I was 33 years old at the time! The gynecologist prescribed tranquilizers.

Needless to say, I had just about lost all faith in the medical profession by that time, and was about to give up any hope of finding a cure for my ills, when I found a copy of *Look Younger and Live Longer* by Gayelord Hauser. Hauser had one piece of advice for a wide array of physical ailments, from wrinkles to rickets: stop eating "dead foods." By dead foods Hauser was referring to refined and processed foods, refined sugar, white flour, coffee and chocolate. His dietary regimen involved eating lots of live foods, such as fresh vegetables and fruits, whole grain breads and cereals and wheat germ, and drinking herbal teas and water.

I could easily recognize myself as a dead foods addict. As a girl, I had prided myself on my cake-decorating ability, and I was always making and eating pastry, fudge and other desserts. Our family meals had two or three starch dishes at a time. The coffee pot and the plate of sweet rolls are common sights in police stations, courthouses and offices, and ours in Akron was no exception. I learned later that I have a brain allergy to caffeine; in 1963 I was drinking 10 or 12 cups of coffee a day. The idea that my bizarre symptoms could be caused by dietary deficiencies or excesses seemed to make sense — at least, more sense than anything I heard from the medical community.

I decided to take Hauser's advice. I gradually began to get off caffeine by cutting my regular coffee with decaffeinated until I could do without it entirely. I stopped eating white flour products and sugar, and replaced them with natural foods which Hauser recommended. It was not an easy transition to make at first, especially with a small child in the house. But I stuck to it and made the change.

It worked — and how it worked! I began to get a good night's sleep every night, and woke up feeling refreshed. My nightmares disappeared, as did my cold sweats and mental lapses. I found I had an unlimited store of energy to draw on, and I was able to get more work done and more enjoyment out of play. My health improved more than I could have expected. And the best thing was that I didn't have to wait — in a matter of weeks I felt like a completely different human being, a brand new creature!

As with anyone who is the recipient of a miracle, I began to feel a bit apostolic. I felt that if a mere change in diet could make such broad and significant changes in my life, the nutritional approach should be able to help anybody. I started to pay attention to the eating habits of the probationers who came through my office. That's when I made the real breakthrough.

I discovered that a huge proportion of the people who were getting into trouble were junk food junkies. Many were alcoholics or heavy drinkers, and were simultaneously living on booze and sugared snacks. The connection seemed obvious to me: If these men and women were living on processed foods and snacks, how could they get any nourishment? If they were undernourished, how could their central nervous systems be functioning properly? Finally, if their brains and nerves were malfunctioning, how could one expect them to behave sanely in society?

I came across a little booklet which seemed to confirm my suspicions. Entitled *Low Blood Sugar,* it detailed the disorder known as hypoglycemia and gave a list of its symptoms. I immediately recognized many of them as problems common to my probationers: irritability, uncontrollable thoughts and emotions, a "short fuse," depression and suicidal tendencies, insomnia and phobias, violence and aggression. I copied the list and began giving it as a questionnaire to my subjects. Out of a list of 93 symptoms, I discovered that most of my subjects complained of 30 or 40, and sometimes as many as 60 to 70. The minimum score needed to pinpoint hypoglycemia is 25.

I did not have many restrictions placed upon me in my work; I was expected by the judges to keep my charges out of the courtroom, and any legal way I could find to do that would be fine with them. So I began using the diet and encouraging people. At that point I was just testing isolated individuals whom I knew to be in particularly bad shape. But before too long I was using the techniques on everybody.

Instead of sending my subjects off immediately to a psychiatrist, I placed them on the diet I found in the *Low Blood Sugar* booklet. It consisted of a total ban on sugar, white flour products, chemical additives, caffeine and alcohol, and emphasized the consumption of fresh fruits and vegetables, whole grains and such lean meats as chicken, veal and fish, and plenty of water. I also discovered that many of my subjects had dangerously high levels of toxins such as lead and cadmium in their blood, and I learned that these toxins could cause emotional and behavioral disorders. These people I referred to the Baron Clinic for testing and chelation therapy. The personal counseling came later.

My success surprised even me, not to mention my probationers. They could hardly believe how good they felt, how calm, how energetic and alive. An incredible number of them managed to stay on the straight and narrow and out of the courtrooms. By this time I had become head of the Cuyahoga Falls Probation Department, and a common refrain in the courtroom was, "Your honor, I really believe I won't be getting into trouble anymore. Mrs. Reed has me on this diet..." It wasn't long before the judges began to sense the effectiveness of this approach, of getting the body healthy before working on delinquent behavior. By 1973, one of the judges I worked with got into the habit of saying "I'm going to send you down to Barbara Reed, and you're going to stay on the diet she gives you. If you don't, you'll be back in trouble — and next time you're going to jail!"

Word of my success began to spread. One day I got a call from Timothy Shellhart of the Wall Street Journal. Shellhart was working on an article about the connection between diet and criminal behavior. He had gotten in touch with the Huxley Institute for Biosocial Research in New York, which had just sponsored a seminar at which I had presented the results of my program. Huxley Institute referred Shellhart to me. I spoke with him for awhile, and he seemed enthusiastic. But months passed, and no article appeared.

Finally, on June 2, 1977, the piece hit

the front page of the Wall Street Journal, and my life has not been the same since. The next day I was contacted by CBS News, which wanted to do a story on my work. The folks I worked with in Cuyahoga Falls knew that I was an effective probation officer; but when those camera crews rolled into the building, heads turned! Of course, my newfound celebrity status was very flattering, but more exciting were the contacts I made. Dozens of people in various professions had made the connection between diet and behavior, but they had never been taken seriously until my story appeared. I even learned a name for our discipline — orthomolecular psychiatry, which meant concentrating on the biochemical molecular processes in the central nervous system.

Since then I have made many talk-show appearances and news of my work has been published in many periodicals. Perhaps the most rewarding experience, though, was my opportunity to testify before Senator McGovern's Select Committee on Nutrition and Human Needs. The senators were very interested in what I had to say; they could see the implications for the federal courts and penitentiaries, not to mention the health and well-being of all Americans. The committee included my suggestions in its report and recommendations. I also testified before a legislative committee in Los Angeles County. As a result, all junk and processed foods have been removed from Los Angeles juvenile correctional facilities.

My message everywhere has remained the same: A simple diet of whole foods, eaten as fresh, unprocessed and pure as possible, is absolutely necessary in order to give the brain and the rest of the central nervous system what it needs to function properly. On the other hand, ignoring the nutrition of the body is the most dangerous mistake one can make. A malnourished central nervous system will inevitably lead to serious physical and behavioral problems, problems which no amount of medication or psychiatry can touch. I urge parents of delinquent youngsters, or those who want the children of today to avoid becoming the criminals of tomorrow, to read this book carefully, and pay heed to its advice.

I don't want to claim that a whole foods diet is the cure for every type of emotional, psychological and behavioral disorder. Certainly all that mainstream psychiatry and counseling have to offer must be taken into account. But trying to correct a person's misbehavior before he or she has an adequate diet is very much like trying to ride a bicycle without filling the tires with air, or driving a car without first putting in gasoline — it won't, it *can't* work.

It is especially the parents of young people who ought to be concerned with this. Almost every parent wants a better world for his or her children than the one we find ourselves in today. The rise of crime and violence, the abuse of women, children and the elderly make us all wonder if there *will* be a world for the young generation to inherit. What is important for parents to know is that by doing something very basic and simple — by making sure that your kids are well nourished — you can make progress toward solving the problems of criminality, delinquency, violence and mental illness, and even help reduce the tremendous toll that crime and the rehabilitation of convicts takes on the resources of society.

Raymond and Ruth are a good example of how young people respond to this simple therapy. I advised them both to go on the diet. Raymond responded enthusiastically. His girlfriend's response was less impassioned. She stayed on the diet a little while, cheating constantly, and finally let it lapse altogether. She became so resentful of Raymond's progress that she actually refused to cook the whole foods his diet required. Their relationship ended soon after, and she has since been arrested three times.

Raymond, on the other hand, is in

much better shape. His parents noticed an improvement in his behavior and attitude within a week after he started the diet. Raymond was amazed at his own new energy level, which increased so that he could pursue many projects. He found it easier to do his job, and his fellow employees have commented on his dedication and enthusiasm. His crying spells, once an almost constant occurrence, gradually lessened and stopped, and his self-destructiveness ended. Instead of feeling suicidal, he has a positive zest for life. Raymond bears little resemblance to the would-be murderer I first met.

The future is not nearly so bright for all those who have been so morally and emotionally decayed that they try to kill somebody. Another would-be slayer, more notorious than Raymond, is a case in point. Twenty-five-year-old John Hinkley Jr. is sitting in a Washington, D.C. mental institution as of this writing, convicted of the attempted assassination of the President of the

United States — an act he thought would impress a young and famous actress. Friends of Hinkley say he was a junk food addict, that his apartment was littered with debris from fast-food restaurants. Testimony from the trial shows that Hinkley had been eating at a McDonalds a short while before he tried to kill the President. While Hinkley will no doubt receive a full battery of mainstream psychiatric treatments, the chances that his metabolic and nutritional background will be evaluated are slim. Right now, it appears John Hinkley will spend the rest of his life in a mental institution.

CHAPTER TWO
THE BIOCHEMISTRY OF CRIME

The functioning of the brain is dependent on its composition and structure; that is, on the molecular environment of the mind.

— *Linus Pauling*[1]

No twisted thought without a twisted molecule.

— *R.W. Gerard*[2]

"You are what you eat." The phrase is so common to us now that we overlook its deeper truth. Human behavior is rich, complex, and often mystifying; but when we trace an action down — down through organ systems to organs, to cells, to the dizzying array of amino acids, enzymes, neurotransmitters and even beyond — we arrive in the end at a basic denominator: the action and reaction of molecules.

The chemical components of our bodies, substances as familiar as oxygen and as obscure as 3-hydroxyanthranilic acid, are responsible for every function and action. Molecules make up the cells which are the building blocks of organs; molecules provide the fuel which the cells need to carry out their work; molecules help the energizing process take place. The beat of the heart, a twinge of pain, a loving touch — all are, at their root, molecular reactions.

And there is only one source of these molecules or their building blocks, the interactions of which make up our very lives: our diet.

Every protein in the body, every bit of fuel in the blood, every enzyme necessary for the thousands of reactions that take place every second, come directly from or are derived from what we eat. When we understand this, the equation becomes simple: If, through diet, we provide our bodies with the proper molecules in the proper amounts, our bodies will function normally. If, on the other hand, our diets do not provide the cells with the substances they need, our bodies will malfunction in one way or another.

In this chapter I will discuss the role of improper diet in the malfunction of one organ in particular: the brain.

It is the human brain which has placed our species at the top of the evolutionary ladder. It is indeed an amazing piece of equipment. It is built of thousands upon thousands of components, arranged in complex patterns whose importance in the thought process we are only beginning to understand. Each cell communicates with the others with electrical and chemical signals of incredible delicacy. The brain is able to monitor and to some extent control a vast number of metabolic functions, while at the same time enjoying (or composing) a symphony, reading a book, following an argument or making sense of a recipe. It is the most important organ in the body; every other part may be removed or replaced, but shut off the brain and you have killed the organism.

Paradoxically, perhaps, the brain is not only the most important organ, but the most vulnerable as well. Because of the precise specialization of each cell, the brain lacks many of the self-defense mechanisms present in the lesser organs. It can store no energy, it can survive only a few minutes without oxygen and it decays very rapidly under adverse conditions. When something is wrong with the body, the brain suffers first.

Because the brain is so vulnerable to its molecular environment, it is the most directly affected by diet. Thus we would expect that the visible consequence of brain function — behavior — will be strongly influenced by diet. In the rest of this chapter we will explore this diet-behavior link in greater detail.

Hypoglycemia

Energy, of course, is what makes the body run. This is true for the brain as well. Energy is not only required for the electrochemical signals that pass from cell to cell, it is also needed to keep the cells alive, to build new cells and to record the information which continually bombards the senses. Without a steady supply of enough energy, the brain cells stop working and soon they begin to die.

The fuel used by brain cells is called glucose, or blood sugar. In order to work properly, the brain cells need a steady supply of blood sugar. The body makes glucose out of carbohydrates from the food we eat. There are two kinds of carbohydrates: sugars (or simple carbohydrates) and starches (or complex carbohydrates). If the body has used up its supply of carbohydrates, it can make blood sugar out of glycogen, an energy storage product kept in the liver and muscle tissues. Furthermore, if the body's store of glycogen runs out, it can even convert protein and fat into glucose. The fact that the body has all these fail-safe devices is a sign of how important a stable supply of blood sugar is for the brain and the rest of the body's cells.

Many Americans however, can't count on this stable supply of glucose. Instead, their blood sugar levels are too low to meet the brain's needs. They have chronic low blood sugar, or hypoglycemia.

For a minority of these people, the low blood sugar state is caused by damage to or cancer in the glands which produce the hormones which regulate blood sugar. But by far the majority of hypoglycemics are reactive or functional hypoglycemics: In other words, their blood sugar drops as a reaction to the food they eat.[3]

This is not a normal reaction. It is so wide-spread because of a radical change in the diet of Western society, a change which has taken place just within the last eight decades of human history. I'm talking about the revolutionary increase in the consumption of white sugar.

White sugar — sucrose is its chemical name — is a simple, very highly refined carbohydrate. It is extracted from sugar cane or sugar beets. While sugar is still part of a plant it is combined with other nutrients like vitamins, minerals, enzymes and fiber. In the refining process, however, all these other things are simply thrown away. White table sugar is more than 99 percent pure sucrose. This is a much higher concentration of sugar than is found in fruits, vegetables, grains, or any other food in nature. The "purity" of white sugar means it delivers nothing but calories — no other nutrition of any kind.

This purity also means that white sugar enters the blood very quickly. Sucrose is a simple carbohydrate. It's simple because it has just a few atoms in its molecule, so the body doesn't have to do much to break it into glucose and fructose, which are even simpler. As a result, much of the sucrose a person eats gets into the bloodstream shortly after reaching the intestines. Starches, on the other hand, have many more atoms in complex arrangements, so these complex carbohydrates must be broken down more slowly.

Secondly, unlike the sugar found in fruits and vegetables, white sugar is not combined with fiber. Fiber is a tough, chewy plant substance which does not break down in the stomach. This means two things. In the first place, large quantities of white sugar can be consumed much faster than sugar in the natural state. For instance, you would have to eat four large apples — more than a pound — in order to consume the quantity of sugar found in two ounces of peppermint candy.[4] Few people are ravenous enough to eat that many apples in a sitting, yet it is easy to eat a handful of mints without even thinking about it.

Furthermore, in the digestive tract, fiber remains intact and helps digested food move without becoming sluggish and compacted. Fiber limits the amount of sugar that can be absorbed in the intestine by keeping some of it from touching the intestinal wall. Fiber-bound sugar is absorbed more slowly than refined sugar in the same way that a bowl of peanuts in the shell are eaten more slowly than shelled peanuts — you have to get the shells out of the way. Nothing stands between refined sucrose and the intestinal wall, so it is absorbed quickly.

Because our bodies have not adapted to the fast absorption rate of refined sucrose we cannot use it properly. When you eat white sugar, or a food rich in sucrose, virtually the entire sugar load enters the bloodstream within a few minutes. The blood glucose level jumps very quickly. The body isn't expecting the jump — instead it's looking for a gradual gentle rise in serum glucose. Consequently it responds by producing insulin in the pancreas. Insulin acts to take the excess glucose out of the bloodstream and store it in the liver as glycogen. But because the climb in blood sugar is so great, so swift, the pancreas over-reacts and floods the system with more insulin. More and more glucose is taken out of the blood until the sugar level is drastically low. The most obvious symptom of this low blood-sugar state is hunger; the body calls for food, desperate to raise its glucose levels back to normal. Unfortunately, this often means the individual craves something sweet. If the person eats something with sugar in it, the reactive hypoglycemic cycle starts all over again.

This rocketing/plummeting blood sugar syndrome is an insult, a shock, to the entire system. If it were a rare occurrence, however, the body would be able to recover and eventually establish a normal glucose level. But for most of us the hypoglycemic cycle isn't a rare metabolic crisis; *it is a way of life.*

At the beginning of this century, the average consumption of white sugar was about four pounds per person per year. Some researchers have suggested that, even at this level, our young love affair with sucrose was beginning to take its toll on our mental and emotional health[5]. But today our sugar intake has increased 2,500 percent to over 129 pounds per person per year![6]

Every time I mention that ghastly statistic, I am met with disbelief. People simply can't imagine how they could eat 100, 200, even 300 pounds of sugar a year. "How can that be?" they ask, "I only use a few teaspoons a day!" But the truth is that only a small proportion of our daily sugar consumption comes from the sugar bowl. The majority of it — 70 percent, in fact — comes in prepared, processed foods.[7] Over the last several decades the food industry has been steadily increasing the amount of sugar it puts in foods — primarily to encourage overconsumption.[8] The sugar content of the foods we eat every day is truly staggering. Del Monte canned peaches in heavy syrup are 12 percent sugar by weight, General Foods' Tang and Jello are 13 percent sugar, Morton's Coconut Cream Pie is 24 percent sugar and many kids' breakfast cereals contain nearly 60 percent.[9]

When figures like these are converted into more common measurements the results are truly amazing. We may limit ourselves to a teaspoon or two of sugar in our morning coffee, but do we realize that the 16-ounce Coke we have for lunch contains *twelve* teaspoons? Similarly, two ounces of Kellogg's Sugar Smacks, a doughnut, a chocolate bar or a cup of chocolate milk contain about four to seven teaspoons of sugar. Even a diminutive stick of gum can contain ½ teaspoon of sugar — about equivalent to one sugar cube.[10]

Even many foods which we don't think of as "sweet" can contain a lot of sugar. Gerber Plums with Tapioca baby food contains more than 13 percent sugar, tomato catsup may contain up to 29 percent sugar, Shake 'n' Bake is 39 percent sugar, and even the salt used in some fast food restaurants contains 30 percent sugar. Many medicines are heavily laden with sugar: Hold 4 Hour Cough Suppressant is 62.4 percent sugar, Regular Flavor Listerine is 68.9 percent, and Chewable Chocks vitamins are 55.9 percent sugar.[11] Since our consumption of products like these is rising steadily, it's not hard to see where our massive sugar intake comes from.

Because we eat so much refined sucrose, then, our endocrine systems are constantly shocked. The pancreas produces more and more insulin as soon as it senses sugar in the blood, because it comes to expect an overload. The blood sugar lifts get higher, the drops get lower. When the endocrine system is always operating on this sugar-stress hair trigger, the inevitable result is frequent low blood sugar — or reactive hypoglycemia. And with most of us packing away hundreds of pounds of sucrose a year, it is not at all surprising that as many as 50 percent of all Americans may be hypoglycemic.[12]

This lack of blood sugar starves every cell in the body, leading to a general feeling of weakness. But the cells of the brain are especially starved. As the blood sugar drops, the cerebrum — *the area of the brain responsible for thought, learning, and moral and social behavior* — starts to shut down, and the brain diverts its dwindling energy resources to the brain stem, which controls the more primitive responses: the drives for food and sex, aggressive/defensive instincts, basic bodily functions, etc. Individuals in a hypoglycemic state thus exhibit apprehension, trembling, sweating, vertigo, loss of coordination, irritability, confusion and amnesia.[13] In severe hypoglycemia, these symptoms may be a prelude to complete blackouts — long periods of time in which the person walks and talks and may appear perfectly normal, but from which they awake with no memory of what went on.

Hypoglycemics may also experience bizarre hallucinations and other severe sensory distortions. One probationer of mine, a hypoglycemic, aggravated his condition on the night of his arrest by drinking alcohol, which functions in the body as a sort of super-refined carbohydrate to provide a faster lift — and a sharper plunge — than even sucrose. Within minutes of taking a drink, this man got the sensation that the people around him were very tiny. At the same time they seemed very close to him, and yet somehow oddly distant. Frightened, he ran from the bar. Two people noticed his alarming behavior and tried to stop him from roaring off in his car. He almost ran them over.

The average psychiatrist would diagnose these mental dysfunctions not as hypoglycemia, but as neurosis, psychosis or schizophrenia. Indeed, the connection between low blood sugar and mental illness is fairly well established. As early as 1935, researchers like Dr. M.S. Jones, then assistant physician at the Royal Edinburgh Hospital for Nervous and Mental Disorders, were noting the drastic emotional effects of low blood sugar and stating, "Such complaints...may easily be diagnosed as being due to an anxiety neurosis, hysteria or neurasthenia (a neurosis characterized by chronic abnormal weakness)."[14]

Jones related the case of one 36-year-old woman who was hospitalized after five years of vomiting after every meal. The woman was subject to "hysterical attacks, during which she became extremely weak, somewhat incoherent, emotionally unstable, and would throw articles at her husband." She was given a Glucose Tolerance Test (see Chapter Three) and found to be hypoglycemic — a diagnosis confirmed by the fact that her violent spells were nearly always accompanied by a craving for sweets.

Since the thirties the coincidence between hypoglycemia and mental illness has been thoroughly documented. Doctors Wendel and Beebe noted in 1973 that neurotics and schizophrenics who tended to suffer anxiety were more likely to be hypoglycemic than were normal subjects.[15] The same workers reported that of 133 studied psychiatric patients, fully 74 percent were hypoglycemic.[16] Similarly Robert Meiers estimates the prevalence of relative hypoglycemia among schizophrenics to be about 70 percent.[17] The hypoglycemia-mental illness connection is further confirmed by the fact that dietary correction of hypoglycemia very frequently lessens or reverses neurotic, psychotic and schizophrenic symptoms (see Chapter Five).

The relationship between low blood sugar and mental illness has a direct bearing on the diet-crime link. Many of the probationers I see have long histories of medication and/or hospitalization for psychiatric disorders. When a schizophrenic commits a crime, it is frequently quite bizarre, because the act springs from perceptual changes and delusions far removed from the real world.[18]

Mental illness, then, is one intermediate factor linking diet to crime. Another is alcohol abuse. As we noted before, alcohol affects the metabolism much like a highly refined carbohydrate — it has fewer carbon atoms per molecule than sucrose, so it enters the bloodstream quickly, often directly through the stomach lining. It is thought that hypoglycemics may turn to alcohol as a way of lifting blood sugar levels more quickly. While the relationship is difficult to recreate in a laboratory, collected evidence strongly supports the contention that alcohol addiction can be a symptom of hypoglycemia. For instance, researchers at Loma Linda University, working under Dr. U.A. Register, have been able to induce craving for alcohol in rats by feeding them a diet high in sucrose.[19]

Further evidence is provided by the fact that the majority of alcoholics are hypoglycemic. Researchers Poulos, Stoddard and Carron began a study of 200 alcoholics in 1973. Ninety-seven percent of this group were found to be hypoglycemic, as opposed to 18 percent in a control group.[20] Dr. R.O. Brennan quotes one psychiatrist who proclaimed, "I have examined hundreds of patients, and found that every alcoholic tested had hypoglycemia."[21] I can only add that my own experience with hypoglycemic probationers has been very similar. There is of course a "chicken-and-egg" dilemma here, since high alcohol consumption usually causes changes in dietary habits which in themselves aggravate hypoglycemia. Yet the exciting success that physicians report when they treat alcoholics for hypoglycemia (as high as 71 percent sobriety, as compared to 25 percent for groups like Alcoholics Anonymous[22]) seems to demonstrate that low blood sugar is at the root of this insidious chemical dependency.

Once again, the alcohol-diet connection is of interest in this discussion because of the high rate of alcohol abuse among criminals.[23] Criminologist Alexander Schauss reports that in his study of over 1000 juvenile defendants, over half were arrested while under the influence of alcohol.[24] The National Institute of Alcohol Abuse and Alcoholism estimates that 29 to 40 percent of all accident, homicide and suicide fatalities are indirectly caused by alcohol[25] — and even this figure may be too conservative. If diet can drive you to drink, then, it stands a good chance of driving you to crime as well. If the only adverse effect of low blood sugar was increased alcohol consumption, that alone would be enough to make it an important contributor to crime and delinquency.

But hypoglycemia has another

symptom which far more directly contributes to aberrant behavior: increased aggression. Recall that in times of stress we show two different kinds of reactions. There are the primitive "fight or flight" reactions, and, at a higher level, more reasoned and socially-formed stress responses. For example, if we argue with someone, the "gut level" messages being sent from the brain stem may tell us to hit the person. The higher brain, on the other hand, may, as the seat of our social conscience, caution us that violence is an unacceptable method of resolving conflict, and prompt us to seek a more peaceful outcome. But in a hypoglycemic state, it is precisely these "socially responsible" areas of the brain which have shut down because of lack of energy or are otherwise malfunctioning. Only the more primitive, more aggressive brain stem is in operation. Thus the person in a low blood sugar state cannot respond to a stress situation in a constructive, socially acceptable manner.

As we've already seen, aggressive or

violent behavior has long been associated with the symptomology of hypoglycemia.[26] Yaryura-Tobias and Neziroglu have noted that low serum glucose is associated with brain dysrhythmia and aggressive behavior in certain patients.[27] Dr. Robert E. Buckley has also noted this hypoglycemia-aggression link, especially in those who already show temporal lobe dysfunction.[28] University of Nevada researcher Dr. William Hudspeth has indicated that extremely anti-social acting-out behaviors may accompany low blood sugar, and other workers have obtained similar results.[29] [30] [31]

Perhaps the most notorious example of low blood sugar and aggressive behavior is that of the Qolla Indian tribe, which makes its home around the Lake Titicaca region between Peru and Bolivia. California ethnographer Dr. Ralph Bolton has called the Qolla the "meanest and most unlikeable people on earth." Bolton reported that most of the Qolla are continually involved in extremely anti-social behavior, including murder, rape, arson and stealing. Over half the heads of households in one village had been directly or indirectly implicated in a homicide. Their diet? It was high in refined carbohydrates, low in protein and included plenty of alcohol and adrenal stimulants like caffeine. Bolton found that 55 percent of the Qolla were hypoglycemic.[32 33]

The Qolla are simply an extreme example of hypoglycemia-related aggression. Thousands — maybe even millions — of Americans show similar behavioral effects of sugar consumption. We witness it dozens of times every day — the overemotional argument, the pushing, shoving ticket line, the barroom brawl. As someone who works with those in trouble, I see low blood sugar violence constantly. Often an individual will be extremely violent when arrested, and several officers are needed to restrain him. During the first interview, the probationer will often confess that he remembers nothing about the incident.

These people are almost always hypoglycemic or diabetic, and at the time of their arrests they are in a severe sugar low, often made worse by alcohol consumption.

I have dealt with hypoglycemia first in this discussion of the biochemistry of crime because I believe it is the single most important link between diet and delinquent behavior. As we have seen, hypoglycemia is widespread. Its effect on the body — and especially on behavior — is drastic. And, as we'll note later in this chapter, sugar consumption is linked with other nutritional distortions. I am convinced that if we could eradicate hypoglycemia, many other mental illnesses and behavioral disorders would take care of themselves.

Nutrient Deficiency

Besides energy, the brain needs other nutrients. The *macronutrients* serve major functions: Carbohydrates provide fuel, as do fats; proteins are the building blocks of cells, and the components of protein — amino acids — play other important roles, as we shall see. However, there is another class of nutrients which, until recently, have been almost entirely ignored — the *micronutrients*. These are the vitamins, minerals and enzymes. Although they are present in smaller quantities than are the macronutrients, they too have a crucial part to play: they enable every one of the thousands of chemical reactions which take place in the brain to proceed normally. Without them, it doesn't matter if your diet is loaded with carbohydrates, fats and proteins. You will die. If the nutrient supply to the brain is distorted, behavior is distorted.

The range of nutrients with psychochemical importance is broad. According to Dr. Linus Pauling:

> "The proper functioning of the mind is known to require the presence in the brain of molecules of many different substances. For example, mental disease, usually associated with physical disease, results from a low concentration in the brain of any one of the

> following vitamins: thiamine (B1), nicotinic acid or nicotinamide (B3), pyridoxine (B6), cyanocobalamine (B12), biotin (H), ascorbic acid (C) and folic acid. There is evidence that mental function and behavior are also affected by changes in the concentration of the brain of any of a number of other substances that are normally present, such as L(+) glutamic acid, uric acid, and y-aminobutyric acid."[34]

The specific actions of these substances are still poorly understood, and there's no room to discuss them all here. But let's take a look at a few of the most important nutrients, and how they influence behavior.

Amino Acids and Neurotransmitters

The main functional units of the brain are called neurons, and these function interdependently by exchanging electronic signals. Behavior and other body functions are controlled by the way these signals move through the complex arrangements of neurons. Each individual neuron releases its electron signal in response to chemical stimulation; these chemicals are called neurotransmitters. When a neuron sends its signal, it also releases neurotransmitters that stimulate other neurons to fire. Thus the primary functioning of the brain is a complex of chemical and electrical signals. In fact, mental and mood changes can be detected by monitoring the activity of certain classes of neurotransmitters. What are these neurotransmitters, and how are they produced?

One crucial neurotransmitter is serotonin, which appears to play a role in maintaining a positive emotional environment. Massachusetts Institute of Technology researchers have demonstrated that individuals with low levels of serotonin may suffer from depression, insomnia and unusually aggressive behavior.[35]

The body manufactures serotonin from the amino acid tryptophan — a nutrient present in meats and other protein foods. Research indicates that many of the symptoms of low serotonin can be reversed by tryptophan injections.[36]

How can serotonin deficiencies come about? Two principal ways concern us here. First, serotonin deficiencies can be caused by a diet that is poor in tryptophan.[37] There is one tryptophan-deficient food that is becoming especially prevalent in our diet: corn. The American consumption of corn has skyrocketed over the past century. We now consume it in hundreds of ways — corn flakes for breakfast, corn oil in margarine, corn bases in bourbon and beer, corn flour or corn starch in many processed foods. Corn, in fact, has replaced much of the wheat in our diet,[38] even though the latter grain has a more reasonable tryptophan balance. Chronic consumption of a tryptophan-deficient diet could conceivably lead to lowered serotonin levels and consequent depression or anti-social behavior. Fernstrom and his associates have discovered that the quality of a single meal can influence serotonin levels significantly.[39]

A normal serotonin level can be distorted through another dietary practice, a somewhat paradoxical one: the consumption of high amounts of meat. It is true that meat is a rich source of tryptophan, and eating meat does elevate levels of tryptophan in the blood. But scientists have discovered that blood tryptophan does not necessarily translate to brain tryptophan. Transport of amino acids to the brain is competitive; that is, several kinds of amino acids use the same pathway — and they all can't go at once. The more kinds of amino acids in the bloodstream, the less chance that any single one type of them will get to the brain in sufficient quantities. Meat provides tryptophan, but it also provides a range of other competing amino acids. Therefore a diet high in meat does not raise brain tryptophan levels. Diets with balanced amounts of meat and carbohydrate foods like grains and vegetables do contribute greater amounts of tryptophan to the brain.[40]

Another important amino acid which acts as a raw material (or "precursor") for neurotransmitters is tyrosine, which is metabolized into the neurotransmitters dopamine and norepinephrine. Both are important in maintaining proper mental function, and imbalances of both have been linked to schizophrenia and other mental illness.[41] Tyrosine has been used to treat depression.

Yet another important neurotransmitter is acetylcholine. Its precursor is not an amino acid, but a vitamin — choline. Doses of choline or supplements of lecithin (a good source of choline) have been helpful in combating senility and other types of mental decay.[42]

These are just a few of the neurotransmitters that scientists have analyzed. It is interesting to note that sugar consumption may have an impact on the production of neurotransmitters. Too much insulin in the blood stream reduces amino acid levels, thus eradicating the precursors of neurotransmitters like norepinephrine. It's postulated that this is another way in which a diet high in sugar can aggravate depression.[43]

Vitamins

Vitamins are substances that help chemical processes along. While several of these have been found to be extremely important in maintaining proper brain function, it's a bit misleading to talk about the actions of a single vitamin. When we talk about the "action of niacin," for instance, or the "function of ascorbic acid," we have to remember that no vitamin works in a vacuum. Vitamins operate together in complex relationships, many of which we still don't fully understand. We do know, however, that if all essential vitamins are not consumed in balanced amounts the effectiveness of any single vitamin is greatly reduced, if not nullified entirely.[44] This fundamental point becomes important both as we try to understand how vitamin deficiences affect behavior and as we discover how to correct these deficiencies.

One of the most important — and certainly the most talked about — psychoactive micronutrients is niacin, or vitamin B3. Niacin is used by the body in the form of nicotinamide adenine dinucleotide (NAD). The body can make NAD from niacin in the diet, or it can metabolize it from tryptophan through a complex series of steps involving several enzymes.

One of the reasons that we know so much about niacin and brain function is that the niacin deficiency disease — pellagra — is usually accompanied by psychiatric symptoms. Pellagra was a widespread disease in the southern United States around the end of the last century, especially among those consuming large amounts of refined white flour, which contained very little niacin. It is also prevalent in areas where a great deal of corn is eaten. Corn is deficient in the tryptophan from which NAD can be made.

The symptoms of pellagra are known as the "Four D's": dermatitis, diarrhea, dementia and death.[45] The "dementia" include such things as visual changes, hallucinations, vertigo, hyperacute sense of smell, dulled sense of taste, parasthesias (abnormal sensations, such as a burning feeling or feeling as if insects are crawling on the skin), disorientation, confusion, memory lapses, depression, anxiety and fatigue.[46] These mental disturbances almost always respond rapidly to niacin treatment.

Although "enrichment" of many processed foods has guaranteed that few people in this country die of advanced pellagra, doctors are beginning to question whether the emotional and mental malfunctions might appear in people with niacin deficiencies which aren't severe enough to cause the more visible symptoms of pellagra. Such a disease is called *sub-clinical pellagra.* One of the first researchers to note the disease was Dr. T.D. Spies, who mentioned subclinical pellagra in his 1938 paper "The Mental Symptoms of Pellagra." He pointed out that:

> Subclinical pellagrins are noted for the multiplicity of their complaints, among which are many that are usu-

> ally classed as neurasthenic. The most common of these are fatigue, vertigo, burning sensations in various parts of the body, numbness, palpitations, nervousness, a feeling of unrest and anxiety, headache, forgetfulness, apprehension and distractability. The conduct of a pellagrin may be normal, but he feels incapable of mental or physical effort, even though he may be ambulatory.[47]

The startling thing about these symptoms of sub-clinical pellagra is that they are very much like those of schizophrenia — a widespread disease, the victims of which occupy one out of every four hospital beds in the United States.[48] As a matter of fact, the symptomologies are so close that some clinicians don't distinguish between sub-clinical pellagra and niacin-responsive schizophrenia. They call both *metabolic dysperception.*[49]

Can the sorts of deficiences that lead to metabolic dysperception actually exist in this society? Are not most Americans consuming the government's Recommended Daily Allowance for niacin (about 20 milligrams)? If they are, how can any of them be suffering from psychiatric disorders because of niacin deficiency?

The answer to these questions is twofold. In the first place, the levels of nutrients set in the USRDA are intended to prevent fatal deficiency diseases. There is no claim that the USRDA provides *optimum* nutrient levels; in fact, many nutritionists and biochemists claim the USRDA for several nutrients is too low. The fact that the recommended allowance for most vitamins has frequently been revised upward seems to justify this view.

But there is a more fundamental explanation for deficiency diseases in our "well-fed" nation, an explanation which revolutionizes almost everything we know about human nutrition. It is the concept of *biochemical individuality*. Simply put, it means there are no "average" human beings. Instead, each of us is biologically unique. Dr. Roger Williams of the University of Texas, a pioneer in the field of research into biochemical individuality, has demonstrated that virtually everything about us — the size and shape of our organs, the speed of our metabolisms and our requirements for nutrients — can vary enormously from one healthy individual to the next. As Williams has written:

> Each human being possesses a highly distinctive body chemistry. While the same physical mechanisms and the same metabolic processes are operating in all human bodies, the structures are sufficiently diverse and the genetically determined enzyme efficiencies vary sufficiently from individual to individual so that the sum total of all the reactions taking place in one individual's body may be very different from those taking place in the body of another individual of the same age, sex and body size.[50]

Williams' own analysis makes this very clear, especially in the realm of nutrition. He cites evidence that the normal level of potassium in the blood, for instance, can be four times as great in one normal, healthy person as it is in another. The nutritional requirement for calcium can vary over a five-fold range; the need for various amino acids can be twice as high in one person as in another. Even the need for "popular" vitamins like A, C, D and the B-complex can vary over a four-fold range or wider. Especially interesting for us is the fact that the dosage of niacin needed to prevent pellagra can vary even between individuals of the same body weight.[51]

Given these findings, we would expect certain individuals to have a need for psychoactive nutrients such as niacin that is far greater than would be satisfied by the average American diet; indeed, it is likely that some could have nutritional needs that could not be fulfilled by any diet without the aid of food supplements. In such instances, a person eating a "normal" diet and getting 100 percent of the USRDA for niacin would still suffer a deficiency and would begin to show the behavioral symptoms of subclinical pellagra. This hypothesis has been put forward by many physicians besides Dr. Williams, and certainly the fact that niacin supplementation has helped both pellagrins and schizophrenics back to health seems to lend support.[52]

In certain schizophrenics, low levels of NAD in the brain may be due to something other than dietary deficiency, however. Research suggests that some schizophrenics are not able to turn tryptophan into NAD, because one or more of the enzymes which control this process are blocked. This blockage may have two harmful consequences. In the first place, one major supply of NAD is blocked off. Secondly, all that unused tryptophan does not remain stable; it may change into one of a number of chemically similar compounds called *indoles,* some of which resemble hallucinogens.[53] For such individuals, simply consuming more tryptophan won't help to reverse NAD-deficiency symptoms, and may aggravate them. Only niacin therapy will help restore the balance.

While niacin is one of the most popular of the psychoactive B vitamins, it is by no means the only one. Deficiencies in vitamins B1, B2, B6 and B12 have been linked to depression and other mental problems. Thiamine (B1), for instance, is necessary for turning carbohydrates into energy in the brain. Deficiencies can lead to general debilitation and personality disturbances.[54] Similarly, dietary deficiencies of vitamin B12 can lead to a host of psychotic conditions.[55]

Other vitamins play important roles in brain function. Among the more noted of these is ascorbic acid, or vitamin C. Its function in the brain is not fully known, but it seems to participate in many reactions. Schizophrenics often show vitamin C deficiencies, and are frequently helped by megadoses of this nutrient.[56]

There's one more thing we ought to cover before we end this discussion of micronutrient depletion and abnormal behavior: the sugar connection. We have already seen how sugar consumption leads to hypoglycemia and thus to aberrant and often violent behavior. But sugar consumption can also cause nutrient depletion. How? The most obvious answer is that foods that are high in sugar — processed foods — are often low in vitamins; of course, sugar itself contains no micronutrients. Thus a high-sugar diet is usually a low-nutrient diet.

But there is another factor involved. Sugar contains no nutrients, yet in order to be turned into energy it must use up a wide range of nutrients. If the meal itself is nutritionally poor, the body must remove what nutrition it can from its own stores to metabolize the sucrose. Thus a meal high in refined sugar not only provides little or no nutrition, but actually robs nutrients from the body. So sugar consumption can damage brain function both by causing hypoglycemia and contributing to nutrient depletion. (We might add that what is true for sugar goes double for alcohol; it not only crowds more nutritious foods out of the diet, but it strips nutrients from the body as it is metabolized.)

Allergic Reactions

We normally associate allergies with rather harmless symptoms: rashes, sniffles, runny eyes, etc. Yet as clinicians have known for many years, allergic (also known as "hypersensitive") reactions can bring on a number of disturbing behavioral effects as well. Dr. Theron G. Randolph has demonstrated that food allergies can provoke lethargy, stupor, disorientation, paranoia, delusions, hallucinations, distraction, agitation, rage, panic, convulsive seizures and coma.[57] And these sensitivities need not be to rare or unusual foods; in fact, some of the most common foods in our diet can cause allergic reactions, and researchers have argued that the more common a food is, the more likely it is to cause an allergy!

The mechanisms for allergy formation, and how sensitivities lead to antisocial behavior, are still something of a mystery. Allergies may develop in any individual, to virtually any substance. They can appear and disappear at any time.

Nevertheless, instances of allergy-induced abnormal behavior have been well-documented. Doctors David S. King and Marshall Mandel showed in 1978 that adult subjects were more likely to exhibit central nervous system complaints such as depression, inability to concentrate and anger when exposed to allergy-producing substances.[58] The emotional reactions to allergens are by no means limited to vague feelings of discomfort. Dr. Doris Rapp found that patients with a history of compulsive stealing stayed out of trouble when their allergies were treated, and that when the treatment was discontinued many began stealing again.[59] In one random sampling of more than 50 patients hospitalized for schizophrenia, more than 92 percent were allergic to one or more common substances.[60] Mandel tested a group of neurotics who had not responded to standard psychiatric treatments, and learned that 88 percent were allergic to wheat, 60 percent were allergic to milk and 50 percent were allergic to corn.[61]

Moreover, allergic reactions often work together to distort behavior. Mandel relates the case of a 40-year-old man who had become a wreck; he had a history of continual fatigue, confusion and nervous tension. A wide range of allergy testing revealed that the man was hypersensitive to a number of substances. For instance, wheat made him nervous and tense, coffee made him lightheaded, chicken made him confused and eggs made it difficult for him to concentrate.[62] It is likely that many people have more than just one allergy with psychiatric consequences; these would be difficult to isolate without careful testing, and that is perhaps why the link between allergic reaction and unusual behavior is so frequently ignored by physicians and psychiatrists.

Most people don't realize that allergies are often marked by an addiction to the reaction-causing food. In some instances a craving for a food may in fact be a symptom that one is indeed allergic to it. As the individual consumes a lot of food, allergens build up in the bloodstream and body tissues. The substances may disturb body function — yet the body has a remarkable way of adapting to such environmental challenges. For some people, this adaptation may go so far that their bodies become accustomed to the offending substance; they must have it, or they develop withdrawal symptoms. This kind of dependence is called a *maladaptive reaction* — the body learns to "need" a substance which is actually harming it. So people suffering from allergies are in a double bind. Either they consume the substance, often in large doses, and experience the tension and hyperactivity exposure can bring, or they go "cold turkey," and suffer depressive symptoms as the body cries out for the allergen to which it has developed a maladaptive addiction.[63]

Since all allergic reactions to food often require the build-up of allergens in the body, it follows that the more frequently a person eats a certain food, the more likely that person is to develop a sensitivity to it. So it's no surprise that the most prevalent foods in a society's diet are the ones which produce the most allergies. In the United States, for instance, the most common allergies are to wheat and corn, followed by coffee, milk, egg, potato, orange, beef, pork, yeast, beet, cane, tomato, peanut and soy. While our diet once contained a wide variety of foods, most of our meals now are made up exclusively of selections from the above list. You'll notice, by the way, that the list contains not a single green or leafy vegetable while it does contain the two sources of white sugar, cane and beet.

One dramatic case of mine illustrates how such allergies work. This man had threatened to murder almost everyone he knew — his girlfriend, his girlfriend's parents, even *his* parents. I met him after he had been arrested on a firearms violation and was put on probation.

This individual showed symptoms of depression, and had suffered from bleeding ulcers since age 15. His aggressive behavior, depression and ulcers were telling signs. "Do you drink a lot of milk?" I asked him.

"Sure," he said, "about a gallon a day."

I told him that his frequent consumption of milk probably meant he was allergic to it. He said he didn't think so; if he didn't drink milk, especially in the morning, he suffered severe stomach pain and retching. He was sure that it was the ulcers that caused his pain, and that the milk somehow soothed them. He didn't relate his aggressive behavior to the pain-milk drinking cycle.

I suspected that the pain and retching in the morning were not caused by nagging ulcers but were withdrawal symptoms which came from spending the night without milk. I convinced him to try doing without the milk for a while.

He experienced some discomfort at first, but after four days his condition improved, and he began to realize that the milk was causing his gastric problems, not curing them. After six days I urged him to try a little experiment — he drank two glasses of milk. As I expected, the pain and vomiting returned shortly after the re-introduction of milk. After three weeks the man had an experience which overcame the last of his skepticism. He tried a bowl of natural ice cream for the first time — and his pain returned. He was a little surprised; this had never happened to him after eating *ice cream* before. The reason? The natural ice cream contained real cream — unlike most other commercial ice creams. After getting this unexpected evidence, he got off the milk for good, convinced that he was allergic. His stomach problems ceased.

But the change in the man's behavior fascinated me more than the relief from his physical ailments. He became a transformed person. After giving up milk he changed from a threatening, vindictive, aggressive menace to a relaxed friendly young man. Today he needs no complex biochemical explanations to convince him of the link between allergies and aggression. He is himself living proof.

We noted above that cane and beet can very frequently cause allergic reactions. For some people, then, cane and beet sugar can do more than bring on hypoglycemia; sucrose can also quickly cause sharp allergy symptoms. One can usually tell the difference between the two kinds of sugar reactions, because hypoglycemia usually takes at least about an hour to set in, while sugar allergies can happen almost immediately.

Another case study will illustrate the sort of behavior sugar allergy can bring on. I once worked with a woman, a former dancing instructor and mother of two, who was showing some disturbing psychiatric symptoms. She was growing very absent-minded, sometimes putting a jar of mayonnaise away with the detergents, sometimes leaving the toaster in the refrigerator. But not all of her behavior could be lightly dismissed. She sometimes screamed wildly and became hysterical with her children. She began to shoplift. Worried about his wife's disintegrating personality, her husband came to me and said, "Something's wrong."

When I suggested there might be problems with her diet, the husband objected. "You've got it wrong," he said, "she's a real health nut. Every night, while I'm eating my steak and potatoes, she's nibbling on this fruit plate she always makes."

It sounded to me as if the woman was eating a lot of sugar — in this instance, fruit sugar. In my interview with her, I showed her a list of foods that were high in natural sugar, and asked her to put a double check mark over the foods she ate frequently during the day. She checked raisins and bananas. I told her that her continual consumption of these foods was overloading her body with sugar, and that to deal with her physical and emotional problems she ought to avoid the fruits and eat a more balanced diet.

She lasted four days on the program, but then broke down and ate a single banana. Within ten minutes she had broken into a sweat, began trembling badly, and felt herself slipping back into one of her semi-hysterical spells. A half-hour later she began to feel better (another sign that her symptoms were not hypoglycemic, but allergic) and she called to tell me she now really believed that it was the high-sugar fruits which were responsible for her problems. She didn't need to try the raisins.

There's another common allergy-producing food that finds its way into sweetened foods: corn. Corn sweetener is replacing sucrose in hundreds of processed foods. While corn sweetener will produce hypoglycemic reactions, just as sucrose will, it is possible that those allergic to corn will also display an allergic reaction to corn-sweetened foods.

There is yet another relationship between sugar, hypoglycemia and allergy. Several researchers have noted that an allergic reaction can cause or worsen a state of low blood sugar.[64] How this happens is not yet completely clear, but there is one possible mechanism which I believe explains the connection, and which also provides a further reason for the extreme addictiveness of allergy-causing foods. The answer may lie in the adrenal glands.

The adrenal glands, located just above the kidneys, are responsible for producing the substance adrenaline. They are triggered by signals from the hypothalamus which is located at the base of the brain. In times of stress, adrenaline helps to convert stored glycogen into glucose, thus raising the blood sugar and producing a burst of energy. An allergic reaction is a stress, and so the adrenals respond by secreting adrenaline. If the body reacts to the resultant blood sugar rise with too much insulin, low blood sugar develops. The individual may wish to raise his or her blood sugar by eating something sweet. On the other hand, the body may remember that eating the allergy-producing food caused an adrenaline rush, and so the person may choose that path to raise blood sugar. If the over-stimulation of the adrenal system continues, the result may be adrenal exhaustion, in which the body can no longer effectively call on its glycogen stores in times of stress, thus leading to a more pervasive hypoglycemic state. While further study of this hypothesis is needed, it seems likely that the allergy-adrenaline-hypoglycemia cycle may explain many puzzling things about the behavior of people suffering from food allergies.

A person can develop allergic reactions not only to foods themselves, but also to the chemicals added to processed foods. There is evidence that such sensitivity to food additives can have a noticeable impact on behavior. The most famous worker in this field was the late Dr. Ben Feingold, who believed that sensitivity to food additives could cause hyperactivity in children. One study conducted by Dr. C. Kenneth Connors indicated that children given an "average" daily dose of food additives in a cookie showed significantly worsened behavior, while children given a similar cookie without additives did not.[65] Many other studies of the behavioral effects of food additives have yielded similar results, although rigorous diet and behavior experiments involving young children are difficult to carry out. The studies showing that children can be allergic to food additives are of vital interest to any parent, but they also concern those of us in the criminal justice system. Research indicates that a high percentage of children judged hyperactive or learning-disabled in elementary school later go on to get in trouble with the law.[66]

We should not rule out the behavorial effect that allergic reactions to food additives can have on adults, however. Although not as much work has been done in this area, at least one study indicates that adults with allergies to some of these chemicals show markedly worsened scores on personality inventories.[67]

Allergies, then, can develop to very common foods, can cause violent behavior, and can interact subtly with our carbohydrate metabolism and with other allergies. With all this in mind, who can truly say how much of the abnormal, aggressive, violent, psychotic or criminal behavior (which some attribute to the decay of our society), might not in fact be due to hidden allergic reactions?

Toxic Substances

So far we have talked about some dietary influences on behavior with which many readers may have been unfamiliar: distortions in the way the body handles sugar, missing psychoactive nutrients, allergic/addictive reactions. There is a more direct way in which our chemical environment — and especially the chemical components of what we eat — can impact on the human mind. This is through exposure to poisons.

Each day we come in contact with hundreds of thousands of substances.

Most of these have been around as long as the Earth itself. Some elements, although they are basic, are now present in our environment in higher concentrations than ever before in the history of the planet. And some are entirely new, artificial substances, the toxicity of most of which is simply not known, and to which our bodies have had no time to adapt. As humanity manipulates its environment more and more drastically, our exposure to chemicals changes in radical and unexpected ways. Let's take a look at just a handful of these substances, and see how they influence behavior.

Toxic Metals

Vitamins are not the only micronutrients; *minerals* also play an important role in the molecular processes which shape our lives. We already know about many of these minerals, such as calcium, which is used in the construction of bones and teeth, or sodium, which is necessary for nerve and muscle function.

One group of minerals are the metals: iron, which helps bring oxygen to the cells; selenium, which, along with vitamin E, helps to slow the aging process; magnesium, which plays a vital role in converting blood sugar into cell energy;[68] and many others.

However, some metals are toxic. They are poisonous because they are antagonists to beneficial minerals; that is, they take the place of nutrients in biochemical functions, thus ruining them. Zinc, for instance, is known to be extremely important in certain brain processes, and recent studies show it is beneficial in the treatment of schizophrenia.[69] Lead, on the other hand, is a zinc antagonist. If there is too much lead and not enough zinc in the bloodstream, lead will take zinc's place in neurochemical functions, with disastrous results. Population studies show that people with a high exposure to lead, either because they live near lead smelting plants, eat lead-based paint, drink water from lead pipes, or live near highways and inhale a lot of automobile exhaust, show increased learning disabilities, increased hyperactivity, and even psychosis in some cases.[70]

Here are some of the more common metals, and the physical and mental symptoms they are known to cause:[71]

Aluminum: Speech disturbance, uncoordination, paralysis, psychiatric disorders, tremors.

Antimony: Loss of appetite, dizziness, fatigue, headache, irritability, abnormal skin sensations, nerve inflammation.

Arsenic: Loss of smell, dizziness, lethargy, abnormal skin sensations, peripheral nervous system disorders, nerve inflammation, weakness.

Cadmium: Inability to smell, fatigue.

Lead: Convulsions, uncoordination, mental retardation, peripheral nervous system disorders, psychiatric symptoms, tremors, visual disturbances, weakness.

Mercury: Appetite loss, speech defect, fatigue, headache, uncoordination, mental retardation, abnormal skin sensations, nervous system disorders, psychiatric symptoms, tremors, visual disturbances and weakness.

Tin: Speech impairment, headache, abnormal skin sensations, nerve inflammation, visual disturbances.

The actions of a person with toxic metal poisoning are often quite bizarre. I once had several probationers who had been arrested for indecent exposure. Their records indicated that they all worked at the same factory — a plant that did a lot of work with metals. Hair analysis (see Chapter Three) revealed that all had acute lead poisoning. Although the connection between lead poisoning and these sorts of sexual misdemeanors is not well-defined, stories like this lead us to question whether the notorious "flashers" have dirty minds, or simply poisoned ones.

A 19-year-old probationer of mine provides a classic case of how an undetected case of metal poisoning can ruin an entire life. The young woman had been arrested for shoplifting, but her problems started much earlier. She was classified as learning disabled as early as the second grade, and had a history of behavior problems. Although she was strikingly beautiful, she saw herself as grotesque. She was a psychiatric mess.

She received a battery of tests at the Baron clinic, from which we learned she was extremely hypoglycemic and had toxic levels of lead and arsenic in her body. Biochemists believe that the highest concentration of lead the body can safely tolerate is 15 parts per million. This woman's lead levels were more than twice that — 37 parts per million!

She was put on a dietary regimen and was given treatments to remove the toxins from her tissues. The woman was extremely uncooperative in the treatments, but still showed encouraging progress. After just a few treatments her lead levels were down to just 11 parts per million. In less than a year her I.Q. scores increased about 30 points. Today she can drive again, is continuing her education, has stayed out of trouble and — best of all — she realizes how beautiful she is.

The depths to which metal poisoning can throw a person is illustrated in another case. This man was a Cleveland dock worker who had been arrested for a drug felony, but managed to get off on probation for a lesser charge.

I have seen few human beings in worse physical condition. When he came to my office he was so weak he could not hold his head up. His hair looked like straw, and I found out he had been losing it by the handfuls for three months. He looked fatigued and uncoordinated. Laboratory analysis of his hair revealed that the man had shockingly high aluminum levels — more than 300 parts per million. Suddenly his poor health and his criminal behavior no longer seemed a mystery to me. The wonder was that he could still walk!

I called the man and his wife into my office, and they sat opposite me holding hands as I told them the news: aluminum poisoning was contributing to the man's personality decay. In our conversation it developed that he had been working at an aluminum smelting plant for the past year, and he began noticing his physical and mental problems after getting the job. He and his wife broke into tears of happiness. The weight of guilt he had been carrying for months slid off. "You see, honey," he sobbed to his wife, "I told you it wasn't me!"

Where do toxic metals come from? Some may come from diet; foods stored in metal containers often pick up contamination. One Consumer's Digest study showed that a majority of canned fruit juices contained high levels of toxic metals.[72] Especially dangerous are foods stored in lead-soldered cans.

Drinking water can be another source of toxic metals, especially copper. A study of the copper content of drinking waters in 27 locations in the Eastern United States revealed that five were at or near the level of copper considered dangerous by the U.S. Public Health Service.[73] In addition, water run through lead pipes is often a source of lead poisoning, as we mentioned above.

There are many other sources of toxic metal exposure: auto exhaust, pollution from smelters and other industries, batteries, fungicides, extra-dry antiperspirants, cigarette smoking (a source of cadmium, lead and arsenic poisoning), soft-drink dispensers and hundreds of others.[74] Alex Schauss has discovered more than two dozen common objects or environments that can be sources of lead.[75]

Another common source of toxic metals in the environment is the burning of coal — something which becomes a greater health hazard as more coal is burned to reduce dependence on foreign oil, while at the same time environmental standards are relaxed. As toxicologist Bernard Weiss so eloquently warns:

> If these issues (involving metal toxicity) seem remote, I urge you to acquaint yourself with recent surveys

> on the impact of acid rain. The unrestricted burning of fossil fuels, especially unscrubbed high-sulfur coal, is accelerating the deposition of toxic metals into soil, waterways and fish at an alarming rate. Vitriolic opposition to environmental controls by electric utilities and local politicians in the midwest may provide temporary financial relief, but it may also spawn many new toxicological and environmental casualties.[76]

It ought to be remembered that, in one sense, toxic levels of lead and other metals in the body can be considered a deficiency disease. Absorption of many kinds of toxic metals can be prevented by sufficient intakes of calcium and iron,[77] as well as vitamins like ascorbic acid (vitamin C),[78] which help remove toxins from the tissues. Furthermore, in many instances toxic metals can only masquerade as their nutrient counterparts when there is not enough of that nutrient present. Even though the toxic metals in your body may be coming from the plant down the street, how they affect you still depends on your diet.

Other Toxins

We have already mentioned the fact that the hundreds of chemical additives we consume in processed food every day can be the cause of allergic reactions, and that such reactions can influence the mind. But some of these additives are dangerous to all consumers. And the ironic thing is that we voluntarily eat several pounds a year of the most harmful of these substances.

A prime example is caffeine. The "lift" that we get from this substance, an ingredient in coffee, tea, cola, chocolate and many over-the-counter drugs, is due to the fact that caffeine stimulates the production of adrenaline. Adrenaline, as we saw, raises the blood sugar level. People who over-consume caffeine, like the young probationers I see who drink a gallon of cola or more every day, are constantly stimulating their adrenal glands. It is only a matter of time before they simply cannot respond to the stresses placed upon them. This adrenal exhaustion means the body can't raise blood sugar when it needs to and hypoglycemia results.

But caffeine has other psychoactive properties. In large single doses it can produce headache, jitteriness and nervousness, and can even lead to delirium. Research indicates that long-term consumption of caffeine in excess of 600 mg. a day (the equivalent of about eight cups of coffee, which is not at all unusual for some of the coffee or cola-guzzling probationers I handled) can cause chronic insomnia, persistent anxiety, paranoia and depression.[79] While some of these symptoms are similar to those caused by adrenal exhaustion, it seems that caffeine has some negative psychoactive properties apart from the havoc it wreaks on carbohydrate metabolism.

Monosodium L-glutamate (MSG) is another common food additive that can adversely affect behavior. Most famous for its use in oriental cooking (the toxic reaction to MSG is known as the Chinese

Restaurant Syndrome), this flavor enhancer is appearing in more and more seasonings and processed foods.

There is much concern about MSG's effects on the central nervous systems of embryos and infants. Writes researcher Charles Nemeroff, "The use of sensitive and specific measures of biochemical constituents in the retina and brain of MSG-treated animals has in almost every case confirmed the deleterious effects of high-dose MSG treatment in the neonatal period." MSG given to embryos and weanling rats causes marked inhibition of neurotransmitter activity, as well as central nervous system damage. When rats receive doses of MSG starting at the first few days after birth, they show less spontaneous psychomotor activity than controls, and do significantly poorer on certain kinds of behavioral tests.[80]

MSG can have adverse effects on older animals as well; for instance, injections into the brains of cats produce EEG seizures, and large doses seem to distort the hormone balances of adult animals. In sensitive human subjects, oral doses of MSG can cause headache, sweating, nausea, weakness, thirst, abdominal pain and other distressing symptoms.[81] While clinical studies have not yet indicated any adverse behavior caused by MSG in adult human subjects,[82] one wonders whether the additive, with its ability to damage the central nervous systems of the very young, ought not to be considered guilty until conclusively proven innocent; there is, after all, absolutely no nutritional justification for the addition of MSG to processed foods.

A brand new additive now on the market is Aspartame, an artifical sweetener being used in some "low sugar" breakfast cereals and pre-sweetened soft drinks. Although Aspartame's producer, Searle, has brought forth a number of studies to show that the sweetener is harmless, Doctors Olney and Reynold have reported that Aspartame can produce lesions in the central nervous systems of young rats. Such evidence was enough to convince the Aspartame Board of Inquiry of the FDA to recommend in September 1980 that the additive not be marketed.[83] However, there is now an ominous "new climate" in Washington, and Aspartame has been cleared for human consumption.

These are just three of the possibly toxic additives which have found their way into our diet. There are thousands of others, and several new additives are developed every year. With the exception of a mere handful, none have been given rigorous testing to determine if they have any long-term impact on the health of the human body and mind. While most are in the "Generally Recognized As Safe" category, one must remember that this judgement is based not so much on medical evidence as on tradition. Claiming an additive is "Generally Recognized as Safe" is tantamount to saying "we've always used it before, and no one's complained yet." Often an additive has been declared safe simply because it was used for many years before the creation of the FDA. Caffeine is a good example. Although it is present in many foods and beverages, and is considered safe by the food industry, many researchers agree that if caffeine were to be developed today, it would be available only by prescription.[84]

So the state of our knowledge about the behavioral effects of food additives is largely a state of ignorance; in some quarters, even willful ignorance. Are these additives necessary? Certainly not. As we shall see in Chapter Four, thousands of probationers, prisoners, mental patients and hyperactive children are right now on diets which completely forbid the consumption of artificial additives — and not a single one has starved; not a single one suffers nutritionally from a deficiency of synthetic chemicals. It occurs to me that glibly condoning the use of worthless additives simply because there is not yet conclusive evidence of their danger is a little like nonchalantly playing Russian Roulette simply because you don't have any evidence that the chamber is loaded.

Our Junk Food Diet — Recipe For Madness

We have seen so far that, for the brain to function properly, it must have the proper molecular environment. The right molecules must be present in the right amounts before those delicate and still mysterious electrochemical reactions, the precursors of thought, may proceed normally. If something happens to disturb the delicate ecology of the brain; if energy supplies are distorted by consumption of sucrose or adrenal overstimulation; if the needed nutrients are missing; if toxic metals are replacing their beneficial counterparts; if the brain is being poisoned — the mind will be disturbed.

The proper molecules — as well as the improper ones — come largely from what we eat. If our diet contains the substances needed for proper brain function, then the brain will work normally; behavior will be rational and constructive, lives will be full and fruitful. If, however, the diet does not supply the proper nutrients, and if it contains harmful substances as well, then the brain malfunctions — and anything from irritability to lunacy may result.

And the alarming point I must make is that *the American way of eating is precisely the sort of diet which will cause brain malfunction.*

What sort of diet am I talking about? I'm talking about a diet high in processed foods, foods that have been altered, sweetened, refined, stripped of nutrients, overcooked, chemically treated. Although the industry which carries out this tinkering with our food supply was almost nonexistent at the beginning of this century, today it is one of the world's largest enterprises, claiming all but 10 cents of our grocery dollar. Thanks to the processed food conglomerates, with their squads of biochemists and millions of dollars earmarked for "research," our diet today bears little resemblance to what we ate just 50 years ago, or indeed to what the human race has eaten for thousands of years.

What is wrong with processed food, and how does it contribute to mental and behavioral disorders?

In the first place, processed foods contain a great deal of sucrose, consumption of which contributes to hypoglycemia, allergic reaction and nutrient loss. Earlier we saw that many foods prevalent in our diet are high in sugar — even those we don't normally think of as sweet. All this hidden sugar means that most of us consume hundreds of pounds of sucrose every year. And this in turn means that we are constantly punishing our endocrine systems, which eventually lose the ability to regulate our metabolism of carbohydrates, and thus to keep the brain well-supplied with glucose. Little wonder that Doctors Cheraskin and Ringsdorf maintain that candy wrappers ought to have the warning "This product can be dangerous to your mental health" stamped on the label, and that an excise tax be placed on junk foods to support the inmates of mental institutions![85]

The food industry adds sugar to its products in order to increase consumption. Sugar is a very addictive substance; the low blood sugar state which you get from eating it makes you crave more. As biochemist and former corporate food scientist Paul Stitt writes in his book *Fighting The Food Giants,* the food industry has noticed that increasing the sugar in a product also increases the amount a person will eat — and that means increased sales.[86] Thus the corporate craving for profits has meant a continual increase in our sugar consumption, so that today sugar provides more calories in our diet than any other source.[87]

Processed food contributes to mental disorder in another way; it is stripped of vital nutrients. The most notorious nutrient-robbing process is the refining of white flour. Whole grain wheat is rich in many vitamins, minerals and other important micronutrients, especially the

B-complex vitamins. In the refining process, however, the outer layer of the wheat berry (called the bran) and the vital heart (called the germ) are discarded, leaving nothing but the starch center (or endosperm). In one process, then, wheat is reduced from one of nature's most nearly perfect foods to one which is nutritionally bankrupt. More than half of each of the most essential nutrients are missing. As Stitt summarizes:

> The milling process destroys 40% of the chromium present in the whole grain, as well as 86% of the manganese, 89% of the cobalt, 68% of the copper, 78% of the zinc, and 48% of the molybdenum. By the time it is completely refined, it has lost most of its phosphorus, iron and thiamine, and a good deal of its niacin and riboflavin. Its crude fiber content has been cut down considerably as well. White flour has been plundered of most of its vitamin E, important oils and amino acids.[88]

So nutritionally poor is refined white flour that the food industry feels compelled to add something to help it masquerade as a food — so they "enrich" it with a handful of synthetic vitamins. Of course, "enrichment" is a cynical term; no attempt is made to restore the full range of nutritional value once present in the whole grain. If someone stole $21 from you, and then, in a fit of remorse, returned $6 or $7, you would hardly feel enriched. Similarly, when the white flour producer removes scores of nutrients and puts back eight, the only thing being enriched is the food industry.

Even after enrichment, white flour contains comparable amounts of only half the nutrients tested for by the U.S. Department of Agriculture that are found in whole wheat bread. Whole wheat contains more than five times the magnesium, three times the phosphorus, twice the copper, three times the zinc and five times the vitamin B6 of white bread. In addition, enriched white bread contains substantially less iron, potassium, pantothenic acid and folacin.[89]

Yet this white flour, as nutritionally

poor as it is, is used in a great number of foods — breads, of course, and buns, rolls, tortillas, cakes, many kinds of candies, gravies, crackers, noodles, pastas, etc. This nutrient-depleted sub-food has been given a prominent place in the American diet.

Processed foods are only pale imitations of the fresh, whole, natural foods our ancestors ate. Many are cooked or prepared under extreme heat, which destroys many delicate vitamins. Others are boiled at some point in their processing, a step which washes out the water - soluble vitamins, including the B-complex vitamins. Almost all processed foods have skin, seeds, pulp or bran removed — and usually these are the parts of food with the greatest concentration of nutrients. What is left of almost every processed food is carbohydrates: either the simple carbohydrates from refined sugars, or highly-refined fiber-free starches, which themselves break down very quickly into glucose.

A quick glance at government nutrition figures tells the whole tale. Canned peaches in heavy syrup, for instance, have just 40 percent of the protein of fresh, raw peaches, and only half the calcium, three-fifths of the iron, about a third of the vitamin A, and around 40 percent of the thiamine, riboflavin, niacin and vitamin C.[91]

Refined cereal products also rate far below their whole-grain counterparts. Sugar-coated corn flakes have only half the protein, 63 percent of the calcium, 42 percent of the iron, 50 percent of the riboflavin, and none of the vitamin A found in whole-grain corn meal.[92]

The more processing done to a food, the more its nutritional profile is degraded. Thus canned tomato soup has just a third of the iron, only three-quarters of the thiamine, 59 percent of the vitamin A and 29 percent of the vitamin C found in whole, fresh tomatoes.[93] Vitamin specialist Earl Mindell reports that processing can destroy pyridoxine (B6), cobalamin (B12), orotic acid (B13), pangamic acid (B15), biotin, pantothenic acid, choline, vitamin E, folic acid, inositol, para-aminobenzoic acid, iodine, selenium and zinc[94] — all directly or indirectly vital in maintaining a healthy mind. Little wonder that Brennan found that the most popular adult diet in the United States was deficient in calcium, vitamin A and the B-complex vitamins.[95]

Besides their high sugar and low nutrient content, processed foods provide a poor brain environment in yet another way — they contain non-nutritive chemicals which may cause allergies or may be toxic. Every year, each of us eats a total dose of about *four pounds* of additives; a huge dose, when you consider that the amount of an additive in a particular serving of food may be just a milligram or two. As we said before, the cumulative effect of all these chemicals is simply not known. Who can predict the behavioral consequences of a lifetime of eating chemical congregations like this:

Bleached flour, sugar, dextrose, corn

> syrup solids, shortening (with antioxidant), leavening, nonfat dry milk, propylene glycol monoesters, mono- and diglycerides, wheat starch, glycerol, artificial vanilla flavoring, guar gum, citric acid and artificial flavoring.[96]

The culprit? A popular cake mix.

Too much sugar, too many possible allergens or toxins, too little nutrition — these are the characteristics of processed food which endanger the ecology of the brain. Inasmuch as almost all of us consume such products every day, each of us stands to suffer from their harmful effects. But there is one group that is more endangered than any other, because this group consumes huge quantities of mind-wrecking junk foods. I'm talking about adolescents.

Adolescents in modern American society are in an unprecedented position. Like all teens everywhere, they face deep changes in the workings of their own bodies and in their relationships with the world around them. But unlike children of other times and other cultures, today's western adolescents wield a great deal of personal power. They have more money, and consequently more advertisers vie for that money. They are more mobile than ever before, many of them owning their own cars. Moreover, they are more independent, eating away from home two or even three times a day. And more than ever, they are eating processed junk foods: donuts and cocoa for breakfast (if they eat breakfast at all); soda, pizza or sandwiches on white bread for lunch; a fast-food burger, fries and cola for supper; candy all through the day. In one survey of 100 teenagers in Ohio, nearly 40 percent said they did not eat breakfast, 54 percent favored sugared soft drinks over milk or fruit juice, and 71 percent liked corn more than peas or broccoli.[97] In a study of Michigan high schoolers, 13 percent showed clear signs of hypoglycemia, and those with family histories of diabetes or hypoglycemia were significantly more likely to drink cola and other soft drinks daily, and to crave sweets, cakes and pastry.[98]

Little wonder that the government's National Nutrition Survey revealed that among a sampled population of adolescents, more than 60 percent were deficient in iron, more than 57 percent did not get enough vitamin A, upwards of 43 percent were deficient in vitamin C, 39 percent deficient in thiamine, 33 percent deficient in calcium, nearly 30 percent deficient in protein, and 16 percent deficient in riboflavin.[99] And while we look at such figures, we ought to recall that they do not tell the whole story. While the diets of most teens are deficient, the nutrient consumption of some is so awful as to make sickness inevitable.

To sum up, then: we know that incorrect nutrition can upset the delicate ecology of the brain, thus leading to neural malfunction and possible antisocial, delinquent or violent behavior. We know as well that processed foods contribute to this chemical brain imbalance. Finally, we have seen that adolescents are eating huge amounts of these junk foods. The argument as I have presented it leads to an alarming conclusion: the rise in crime among teens is, at least in part, due to their consumption of processed foods. Is there any direct evidence to suggest such a link?

There certainly is. Scientific studies and personal observation by myself and other workers in the field indicate that the juvenile delinquent, the convicted probationer and the prison inmate all tend to eat a lot of processed and junk foods, that a great number of these people have hypoglycemia, nutrient deficiencies or allergies as a result of their diet and, most importantly, a majority of them improve and are made healthy, productive members of society when these biochemical imbalances are corrected through proper diet.

The evidence of the diet-behavior link is ample. A study reported in the February 1980 *American Journal of Clinical Nutrition* provides such stark proof of what our children's diet is doing to their minds and bodies that it deserves to be quoted at length.

The study described the symptoms of a group of 20 youths. They exhibited abdominal or chest pains, sleep disturbances, restlessness, walking or talking in their sleep, personality changes, insomnia, recurrent unexplained fever, diarrhea and constipation, chronic fatigue, excessive perspiration, lack of appetite, headache, nausea and vomiting, depression, nasal congestion, coughing, dizziness, difficulty in swallowing, recurrent nightmares, blurred vision and sore throat.

Some of these kids were in remarkably bad shape. One young boy, 13 years old, was the victim of violent, unpredictable mood changes for seven years prior to the study. His stomach cramps were so painful that they were at first thought to be symptoms of appendicitis. In addition he had occasional diarrhea, severe episodes of depression, insomnia and nightmares. Another of the children, a seven-year-old girl, experienced enlargement of the lymph nodes, fever, vomiting and fatigue. She fell asleep at school, sweated excessively and had suffered abdominal pain and constipation since infancy.

What was the link between these children, all of whom had serious physical, mental and behavioral problems? The link was B-vitamin deficiency. They showed the classic signs of beriberi, the thiamine deficiency disease. The vitamin shortage was no mystery, when you consider what the kids ate. They consumed plenty of sugary soft drinks, pastries, candy and snack foods, and got little protein, despite an occasional hamburger or processed-meat sandwich.

According to one of the researchers conducting the study, Dr. Derrick Lonsdale, the children's junk-food diet was producing a state of marginal malnutrition. "I am referring particularly to what dieticians and nutritionists call naked or empty calories — high carbohydrate foods which don't contain any vitamin or mineral supportive qualities at all." Lonsdale pinned much of the blame on soft drinks: "I really believe the most dangerous aspect is the high-calorie drinks they're taking, the carbonated beverages, things like powdered sweet drinks, the fruit drinks. All of these things are being taken by a number of children and adolescents in absolutely fantastic amounts. I think the record I've seen was 98 gallons of cola in two months."

Lonsdale fully affirms the diet-behavior link, based on what he's seen. "Scientifically, we have reason to believe that this approach to diet is changing the balance of neurological transmission which is the hallmark of the function of the brain and the central nervous system. It means that the quality and quantity of nutrition can change your behavior. That's the bottom line."

Lonsdale and his colleague, Dr. Raymond J. Shamberger, found that the combination of refined carbohydrates and thiamine deficiency could have a doubly dangerous effect. "This fact constitutes a difference between our patients and those that might be expected to contract beriberi in a deprived population. It has long been known that a high carbohydrate diet is most dangerous in the presence of a thiamine deficiency...Access to easily assimilable sweet beverages could represent a modern danger which is insufficiently emphasized in American society and may well be responsible for personality traits and symptomatology that are regularly overlooked and considered to be 'the personality of a growing child or adolescent.' "[100]

A 14-year-old male observed by Alex Schauss and Dr. Clifford E. Simonsen vividly illustrates the junk food addiction of many adolescents who get into trouble with the law. This boy had been arrested for vandalism, but it was not his first offense; he had committed two second-degree burglaries in two years. The composite of this young man's diet, which Schauss and Simonsen present, defies belief — and turns the stomach. For breakfast he often ate *five cups* of Sugar Smacks with ½ teaspoon added sugar, a glazed donut and 20 ounces of milk. For lunch he ate two hamburgers, french fries, two slices of white bread, 24 ounces of chocolate milk, and topped it off with two foot-long ropes of red licorice; he might even eat a small serving of green beans. Supper consisted of a peanut butter and jelly sandwich on white bread, a can of tomato soup and ten ounces of Kool-Aid. Throughout the day he snacked on high-sugar foods, and foods with plenty of preservatives and other additives: more red licorice, three beef jerky sticks, a large bowl of ice cream and a very large candy bar.

No one could eat this way and stay sane and healthy. Little wonder, then, that this young man complained of sleeplessness, headaches, nightmares, fainting spells, restlessness, indecision, nervousness, explosive temper and crying spells. Computer analysis confirmed what anybody could have guessed: even though the food he was eating had too many calories and refined carbohydrates, it was woefully deficient in vitamins E, C, B1, B2, B5, B6, B12, para-aminobenzoic acid, biotin, bioflavinoids, selenium and vanadium.[101]

The boy in the Schauss-Simonsen study was eating 36 teaspoons of sugar a day, hidden in the various processed foods he consumed. This may seem amazing to some, but it is a common average dose for kids in trouble. I've seen probationers who consume more than 70 teaspoons of sucrose a day!

In studies of hundreds of young people, the diet-behavior pattern constantly emerges. A study by Dr. Lyelle L. Palmer, for instance, noted that of a group of high-achieving high school seniors, only 2.5 percent consumed high levels of caffeine and sugar, while 37.5 percent of the low achievers were considered caffeine and sugar abusers.[102] A study of 166 women college students showed that 48 percent showed at least two symptoms of vitamin B6 deficiency, 28 percent showed at least two symptoms of vitamin A deficiency, and 21 percent showed two or more symptoms of vitamin C deficiency. All in all, 81 percent showed symptoms of deficiencies in at least two vitamins. Those students who ate the worst were significantly more likely to show psychiatric disturbances than those who ate better.[103]

After reviewing the diets of thousands of probationers, I have seen the following patterns emerge:

1) *No breakfast:* The majority of people I see simply do not eat breakfast. This is a very bad first step, especially for those with distorted metabolism. The body — brain included — needs a good rich source of protein, as well as a good supply of complex carbohydrates, vitamins, minerals and micronutrients after six to ten hours without food. Breakfast primes the entire metabolism for the whole day — eating better later won't make up for skipping breakfast. For hypoglycemics in particular, trying to get through the morning on what's left of the blood sugar after several hours' fast can have troublesome behavioral consequences, as studies with misbehaved schoolchildren indicate.[104]

2) *High consumption of sugar and other refined carbohydrates:* Almost invariably the first thing an offender puts in his or her mouth upon arising is some high-sugar food — cola or other soft drinks, cocoa, sugared coffee, donuts, etc. By this time the blood sugar is often disastrously low, and the hypoglycemic must eat something, *anything,* to get it back up again. Eating sugar sets the individual back in two ways, of course: It starts his or her blood sugar level on the hyper-hypoglycemic roller coaster once again, and at the same time it forces the body to remove nutrients from storage to process the naked calories, thus putting the individual in an even worse nutritional state.

Other refined carbohydrate foods are big favorites with offenders as well. These include white bread, french fries, shakes, spaghetti and macaroni.

We have already noted Dr. Lonsdale's adamance about sugared soft drinks; I can only add my own. For many of the people I see, Kool-Aid and cola are staples. It's not unusual for some of my probationers to be consuming as much as a gallon of Kool-Aid a day; after all, it's cheap and tastes fruity, and of course it's high in sugar. The consumption of sugared soft drinks contributes greatly to the high sucrose intake of probationers.

3) *High consumption of other processed foods:* Even when an offender isn't eating refined carbohydrates, his or her diet is still largely confined to processed foods: canned vegetables (especially corn), processed meats (bologna, hot dogs, etc), pre-packaged entrees, TV dinners and the like. Thus the diet is high in chemical additives and can only do a poor job of replacing nutrients lost because of refined carbohydrate consumption.

4) *Low consumption of lean protein:* As mentioned, the juvenile offender seldom gets the protein needed for proper mental and physical development. What protein foods offenders do eat are generally high in fat: hamburgers, hot dogs, bacon,

pizza. In the rare instances in which they eat chicken or fish, it is almost always deep fried. Such high consumption of fat, much of it saturated fat, stresses the entire body and leads to clogging of the arteries which feed blood and oxygen to the heart and brain. It is estimated that every American over the age of 18 has at least one important artery completely blocked with cholesterol.[105]

5) *Low consumption of fresh fruits and vegetables:* Offenders, especially juveniles, turn up their noses at fresh, raw fruits and vegetables. There seem to be two reasons for this. American culture still presents whole foods as unglamorous and inferior to pizza, Coke and hot dogs. When young people reach for something to eat, they reach for the product that's more highly advertised, more excitingly hyped — and these are the processed foods. Certainly no one is going to spend a lot of money to make some non-patentable food like celery or carrots look flashy.

Secondly, fresh whole foods simply don't have the addictive qualities of processed foods. They don't contain sucrose, salt, fat or chemical flavor stimulants, so they don't satisfy the junk-food junkie's cravings. In this high-tech era in which we've been alienated from our own taste buds, natural foods are something one has to learn to enjoy. Many of the probationers I've seen just haven't learned.

6) *High milk consumption.* We talked about milk allergy/addiction and its behavioral consequences earlier in the chapter. It is true that many of the probationers I've seen drink an amazing amount of milk — sometimes several gallons a day.

Apparently, allergic reaction to milk may be a bigger problem than anyone has yet suspected. The 1978 Schauss-Simonsen study compared the diets of 30 chronic juvenile offenders to the diets of kids who had behavior problems but no criminal background. The comparison revealed one glaring dietary difference: milk consumption. Children who got in trouble with the law drank a lot more milk than those who did not. As Schauss described the results:

> The male offenders consumed an average of 64 ounces of milk a day, while their comparison group only drank an average of 30 ounces daily. Similarly, the delinquent females drank an average of 35 ounces of milk a day, while the comparison group of non-delinquent girls consumed only 17 ounces daily. Among the delinquent boys, two reported drinking more than 113 ounces of milk, or over 14 eight-ounce glasses daily.[106]

But even probationers are not yet at the end of the line when it comes to biochemical degradation. We see the most severe illnesses among the prison inmates. Here a lifetime of poor eating habits is compounded by a state-supplied diet which is notoriously rotten. Thus we find prisoners, many of whom may well have been arrested for dietary-induced behavior in the first place, now becoming even more nutritionally twisted. Studies at the Morristown, New

Jersey, Rehabilitation Center found that prison inmates consume much more refined sugar and caffeine than non-inmates. They discovered that many prisoners were outright sugar addicts, eating the stuff at every opportunity. Little wonder that hypoglycemia rates among inmates run as high as 85 percent.[107]

I have tried to show in this chapter the exorbitant price we pay by ignoring and abusing the molecular environment of the brain. Hypoglycemia, nutrient deficiency, allergic reaction, toxicity; the growing science of neurochemistry demonstrates that all these disorders can affect the way the brain operates, and the way we behave. Further, broad studies and a great deal of clinical evidence indicate that many people who show abnormal, anti-social, delinquent or violent behavior are in fact suffering from brain malnutrition or brain poisoning, possibly brought on by a high consumption of processed food and junk foods. Our rising crime rate must be seen as just another of the health consequences of our love of processed food. Others have documented the links between processed food consumption and cancer, heart disease, diabetes and other killers. I believe, in light of the evidence I have presented in this chapter, confirmed by my years of experience in the criminal justice system, that delinquency, crime and violence must be counted as additions to the list of diseases so miserably prevalent in our over-fed but undernourished society.

The question is no longer, "Is there a diet and crime connection?" but rather, "How long will we let this tragedy continue?"

NOTES

[1]Linus Pauling, "Orthomolecular Psychiatry," in David Hawkins and Linus Pauling, eds., *Orthomolecular Psychiatry* (San Francisco: W.H. Freeman and Company, 1973). p. 2.

[2]R.W. Gerard, in Arieti, S., ed., *American Handbook Of Psychiatry,* Vol. 2 (New York: Basic Books, 1959).

[3]Carl C. Pfeiffer, *Mental And Elemental Nutrients,* (New Canaan, Connecticut: Keats Publishing, Inc., 1975), p. 381.

[4]Calculated from figures taken from A.A. Paul and D.A.T. Southgate, *The Composition Of Foods,* (New York:

Elsevier/North-Holland Biomedical Press, 1978), pp. 194, 242 and United States Department of Agriculture Home and Garden Bulletin No. 72, *Nutritive Value Of Foods,* (Washington, D.C.: U.S. Govt. Printing Office, 1971) pp. 18, 35.

[5]Michael F. Jacobson, *The Changing American Diet,* (Center for Science in the Public Interest).

[6]William Dufty, *Sugar Blues,* (New York: Warner Books, 1976).

[7]Select Committee on Nutrition and Human Needs, United States Senate, *Dietary Goals For The United States,* (Washington, D.C.: U.S. Govt. Printing Office, 1977), P. 48.

[8]Paul A. Stitt, with Mark Knickelbine and Scott Knickelbine, *Fighting The Food Giants* (Manitowoc, Wisconsin: Natural Press, 1980), p. 147.

[9]Jim Hightower, *Eat Your Heart Out* (New York: Crown Publishers, Inc., 1975), p. 79.

[10]Jean Sweet, *The Sugar Case,* (506 Woodside Terrace, Madison, Wisconsin, 1981).

[11]Ira L. Shannon, *Brand Name Guide To Sugar,* (Chicago: Nelson-Hall, 1977).

[12]Dufty, p. 21.

[13]M.S. Jones, "Hypoglycemia in the Neuroses," *The British Medical Journal,* Nov. 16, 1935, pp. 945-6.

[14]Ibid.

[15]Otto W. Wendel and Willard E. Beebe, "Glycolytic Activity in Schizophrenia." in Hawkins and Pauling, *Orthomolecular Psychiatry,* pp. 279-301.

[16]Wendel and Beebe, "Preliminary Observations of Altered Carbohydrate Metabolism in Psychiatric Patients," in Hawkins and Pauling, *Orthomolecular Psychiatry,* pp. 434-451.

[17]Robert L. Meiers, "Relative Hypoglycemia in Schizophrenia," in Hawkins and Pauling, *Orthomolecular Psychiatry,* p. 452.

[18]A. Hoffer, "Mechanism of Action of Nicotinic Acid and Nicotinamide in the Treatment of Schizophrenia," in Hawkins and Pauling, *Orthomolecular Psychiatry,* p. 220.

[19]E. Cheraskin and W.M. Ringsdorf, Jr., with Arline Brecher, *Psychodietetics,* (New York: Bantam Books, 1976), p. 48.

[20]C. Jean Poulos, Donald Stoddard and Kay Carron, *Alcoholism, Stress and Hypoglycemia,* (Davis, California: Davis Publishing, 1976).

[21]Dr. R.O. Brennan, with William C. Mulligan, *Nutrigenetics,* (New York: M. Evans and Company, Inc., 1975), p. 9.

[22]Alexander Schauss, *Diet, Crime and Delinquency,* (Berkeley, California: Parker House, 1981), p. 65.

[23]Russell F. Smith, "Alcoholism and Criminal Behavior," in Leonard Hippchen, ed., *Ecologic-Biochemical Approaches To Treatment Of Delinquents And Criminals,* (New York: Van Nostrand Reinhold Company, 1978), pp. 20-30.

[24]Schauss, *Diet, Crime and Delinquency,* op. cit.

[25]Schauss, *Diet, Crime and Delinquency,* p. 64.

[26]Jones, op. cit.

[27]J.A. Yaryura-Tobias and F. Neziroglu "Violent Behavior, Brain Dysrhythmia and Glucose Dysfunction, A New Syndrome," *Journal of Orthomolecular Psychiatry,* 1975, Vol. 4 No. 4, pp. 182-188.

[28]Robert E. Buckley, "Hypoglycemia, Temporal Lobe Disturbance and Aggressive Behavior," *Journal Of Orthomolecular Psychiatry,* 1979, Vol. 8 No. 3, pp. 188-192.

[29]Schauss, *Diet, Crime and Delinquency,* p. 19.

[30]Brennan, *Nutrigenetics,* p. 122.

[31]J. Kershner and W. Hawke, "Megavitamins and Learning Disorders: A Controlled Double-Blind Experiment," *Journal of Nutrition,* 1979, No. 109, pp. 819-826.

[32]Schauss, *Diet, Crime and Delinquency,* p. 20.

[33]Pfeiffer, *Mental and Elemental Nutrients,* pp. 380-381.

[34]Pauling, "Orthomolecular Psychiatry," op. cit.

[35]Stuart Berger, "What's in Your Food Affects Your Mood," *Chicago Tribune,* July 19, 1982, Sec. 1 p. 13.

[36]John D. Fernstrom, "Nutrition, Brain Function and Behavior," in Sanford A. Miller, ed., *Nutrition & Behavior,* (Philadelphia: The Franklin Institute Press, 1981), pp. 59-68.

[37]Ibid.

[38]Jacobson, *The Changing American Diet.*

[39]Fernstrom, *"Nutrition, Brain Function,"* op. cit.

[40]Ibid.

[41]Alan H. Pressman, "Neurochemistry and Behavior," *The ACA Journal of Chiropractic,* March, 1979, Vol. 13, pp. 15-23.

[42]Fernstrom, "Nutrition, Brain Function," op. cit.
[43]Pressman, "Neurochemistry," op. cit.
[44]R.A. Harte and B. Chow, "Dietary Interrelationships," in M.G. Wohl and R.S. Goodhard, eds., *Modern Nutrition in Health and Disease,* 3rd. ed. (Philadelphia: Lea and Febiger, 1964), pp. 534-544.
[45]A. Hoffer, "Mechanism of Action of Nicotinic Acid and Nicotinamide in the Treatment of Schizophrenia," in *Orthomolecular Psychiatry,* p. 208.
[46]Hoffer, "Mechanism of Action," p. 213.
[47]Spies, T. D., "The Mental Symptoms of Pellagra," *American Journal of Medical Science,* No. 196, P. 4.
[48]Pressman, "Neurochemistry," op. cit.
[49]Bella Kowalson, "Metabolic Dysperception: The Role of the Family Physician in its Diagnosis and Management," in *Orthomolecular Psychiatry,* p. 404.
[50]Roger J. Williams, *Biochemical Individuality,* (Austin, Texas: University of Texas Press, 1977), p. 166.
[51]Williams, *Biochemical Individuality,* pp. 135-165.
[52]Carl C. Pfeiffer and Donna Bacchi, "Copper, Zinc, Manganese, Niacin and Pyridoxine in the Schizophrenias," in Roger J. Williams and Dwight K. Kalita, eds., *A Physician's Handbook on Orthomolecular Medicine,* (New York: Pergamon Press, 1977), pp. 106-120.
[53]Hoffer, "Mechanism of Action," pp. 226-228.
[54]Irmgard Thiessen, "The Role of Thiamine in Research with Animals and in Humans," *Journal of Orthomolecular Psychiatry,* 1978, Vol. 7 No. 2, pp. 107-113.
[55]Antonia J. Deliz, "Large Amounts of Nicotinic Acid and Vitamin B12 in the Treatment of Apparently Irreversible Psychotic Conditions Found in Patients with Low Levels of Folic Acid," *Journal of Orthomolecular Psychiatry,* 1979, Vol. 8 No. 2, pp. 63-65.
[56]Marijan Herjanic, "Ascorbic Acid and Schizophrenia," in *Orthomolecular Psychiatry,* pp. 303-315.
[57]Theron G. Randolph and Ralph W. Moss, *An Alternative Approach to Allergies,* (New York: Lippincott — Crowell, 1980) pp. 138-155.
[58]Schauss, *Diet, Crime and Delinquency,* p. 76.
[59]Doris J. Rapp, "Food Allergy Treatment for Hyper-

kinesis," *Journal of Learning Disabilities,* November, 1979, Vol. 12 No. 9, pp. 42-50.

[60]Cheraskin and Ringsdorf, *Psychodietetics,* p. 130.

[61]Ibid.

[62]Cheraskin and Ringsdorf, *Psychodietetics,* pp. 128-129.

[63]William H. Philpott and Dwight K. Kalita, *Brain Allergies,* (New Canaan, Connecticut: Keats Publishing, Inc., 1980), pp. 23-24.

[64]Marshall Mandel, article in *Journal of the International Academy of Metabology,* March 1975, Vol. 4 No. 1, pp. 83-87.

[65]C. Keith Conner, "Artificial Colors in the Diet and Disruptive Behavior: Current Status of Research," in *Nutrition and Behavior,* pp. 137-143.

[66]Sidney H. Slavin, "Information Processing Defects in Delinquents," in *Ecologic-Biochemical Approaches to Treatment of Delinquents and Criminals,* pp. 75-104.

[67]David S. King, "Food and Chemical Sensitivities Can Produce Cognitive-Emotional Symptoms," in *Nutrition and Behavior,* pp. 119-130.

[68]Earl Mindell, *Earl Mindell's Vitamin Bible,* (New York: Rawson, Wade Publishers, Inc., 1979), pp. 67-96.

[69]Pfeiffer and Bacchi, "Copper, Zinc, Manganese, Niacin...," op. cit.

[70]Pfeiffer, *Mental and Elemental Nutrients,* pp. 311-317.

[71]Adapted from table in Bernard Weiss, "Behavior as a Common Focus of Toxicology and Nutrition," in *Nutrition and Behavior,* pp. 95-107.

[72]*Consumer's Digest.* .

[73]Pfeiffer, *Mental and Elemental Nutrients, p. 331.*

[74]Pfeiffer, *Mental and Elemental Nutrients,* p. 323.

[75]Schauss, *Diet, Crime and Delinquency,* p. 40.

[76]Weiss, "Behavior as a Common Focus," op. cit.

[77]Ibid.

[78]Rhoda Papaioannou, Arthur Sohler and Carl C. Pfeiffer, "Reduction of Blood Lead Levels in Battery Workers by Zinc and Vitamin C," *Journal of Orthomolecular Psychiatry,* 1978, Vol. 7 No. 2, pp. 94-106.

[79]Richard M. Gilbert, "Caffeine: Overview and Anthology," in *Nutrition and Behavior,* pp. 147-160.

[80]Nicholas Freydberg and Willis A. Gortner, *The Food*

Additives Handbook, (New York: Bantam Books, 1982), pp. 556-557.

[81]Charles B. Nemeroff, "Monosodium Glutamate — Induced Neurotoxicity: Review of the Literature and Call for Further Research," in *Nutrition and Behavior,* pp. 177-211.

[82]Ibid.

[83]Ibid.

[84]Gilbert, "Caffeine Overview," op. cit.

[85]Cheraskin and Ringsdorf, *Psychodietetics,* p. 71.

[86]Stitt, *Fighting the Food Giants,* pp. 135-179.

[87]*The Sugar Film,* (Image Associates, P.O. Box 40106, 352 Conejo Road, Santa Barbara, California).

[88]Stitt, *Fighting the Food Giants,* pp. 143-144.

[89]Tom Gorman, "Now we know — wheat does beat white," *Bakery,* June 1981, p. 53.

[90]Figures from United States Department of Agriculture, *Composition of Foods* (Washington, D.C.: U.S. Govt. Printing Office, 1975).

[91]Ibid.

[92]Ibid.

[93]Ibid.

[94]Mindell, *Earl Mindell's Vitamin Bible,* pp. 24-96.

[95]Brennan, *Nutrigenetics,* p. 55.

[96]Michael F. Jacobson, *Eater's Digest,* (New York: Doubleday & Company, Inc., 1976), p. 3.

[97]Louise Fabian, *Teenage Food Survey,* unpublished study, (Girard, Ohio, 1981).

[98]Nola A. Smith, *Investigation of Hypoglycemia as a Causal Factor in Some Kinds of Emotional Distress,* unpublished thesis, Eastern Michigan University.

[99]Senate Select Committee on Nutrition and Human Needs, *Nutrition and Human Needs, Part 3 — The National Nutrition Survey,* (Washington, D.C.: U.S. Govt. Printing Office, 1969), p. 939.

[100]"Junk Foods and a Vitamin B1 Deficiency," *Today's Living,* June 1982, pp. 6-8, 61-64.

[101]Schauss, *Diet, Crime and Delinquency,* pp. 53-55.

[102]Lyelle L. Palmer, "Early Childhood Caffeine and Sugar Habituation," *Journal of Orthomolecular Psychiatry,* 1977, Vol. 6 No. 3, pp. 248-250.

[103]Robert T. Bagley, "Relationship of Diet to Physical Emotional Complaints and Behavioral Problems Reported by Women Students," *Journal of Orthomolecular Psychiatry,* 1981, Vol. 10 No. 4, pp. 284-298.

[104]Cheraskin and Ringsdorf, *Psychodietetics,* p. 122.

[105]The 1977 Working Group to Review the 1971 Report by the National Heart and Lung Institute Task Force on Arteriosclerosis, *Arteriosclerosis,* DHEW Publication No. (NIH) 78-1526.

[106]Schauss, A.G. and Simonsen, C.E., "Critical Analysis of the Diets of Chronic Juvenile Offenders, Part 1," *Journal of Orthomolecular Psychiatry,* 1979, Vol. 8 No. 3, pp. 149-157.

[107]Schauss, *Diet, Crime and Delinquency,* p. 24.

CHAPTER THREE
DETECTING MALNUTRITION

Malnutrition: A state of impaired functional ability or deficient structural integrity or development brought about by a discrepancy between the supply to the body tissues of essential nutrients and calories, and the biologic demand for them.

— The American Medical Association[1]

The well-nourished American is a myth.

— Dr. Carl C. Pfeiffer[2]

Malnutrition. It's a word everyone knows, but few understand.

If I were to ask you to diagnose a case of malnutrition, how would you go about it? Perhaps you would describe the symptoms most commonly associated with starvation: bloated belly, spindly arms and legs, dull eyes. We have all seen the children of poor Third World nations who exhibit these signs, and our hearts go out to them. "If only we could somehow share our superior Western lifestyle with them," we imagine, "how happy they would be!"

As we saw in the last chapter, there are many diseases, mental and physical, that are caused by the supposedly plentiful diet we Americans enjoy. Yet the misconception that malnutrition exists only among the poor and deprived continues, and it has clouded the thinking of the medical and psychiatric communities. The assumption remains that only when a person is literally on the verge of death are we entitled to say that person is malnourished. Therefore we associate malnutrition with those starving children on TV, and never think that we, in one of the wealthiest nations in the history of humanity, could be the victims of a kind of starvation as well.

Hunger researcher Medard Gabel has developed a telling statistic: Ten percent of the world's population are not able to obtain nourishing food. Twenty percent, however, can afford nourishing food but choose instead to buy something under-nourishing.[3] It is not as if these people are deliberately setting themselves up for starvation. But as we have seen, the diets of Westerners are providing fewer and fewer of the micro-nutrients we need to survive and function normally, while at the same time overloading us with fat, refined carbohydrates, salt and chemical additives — and adolescents are most vulnerable in this regard. Teens in America may not be succumbing to exotic diseases like Kwashiorkor or rickets, but their Western style of affluent starvation is taking a terrible toll on their lives — not just in the form of emotional and behavioral destruction, but also as a result of the obesity, heart disease, cancer, diabetes, and diverticular diseases they will begin to suffer as they get older.

The most pernicious, and perhaps one of the most widespread, of these afflictions of Western malnutrition is the psychological one. As I have described in the preceeding chapter, when the body does not have the nutrients it needs to combat stress and continue normal activity, or when the body is loaded down with an overabundance of toxins or refined carbohydrates, the first organs to be affected are the most delicate and complex — the central nervous system and the brain. Such an imbalance contributes to mental problems as minor as lack of concentration, chronic irritability or impulsiveness to disorders as severe as paranoid schizophrenia. And when the central nervous system is not functioning properly, can we expect anything other than abnormal, antisocial behavior?

Therefore, it is important for professionals in the fields of criminal justice, corrections, medicine and psychiatry, and for the general public to realize that our affluent malnutrition does have an incredible impact on our health and behavior. If we are to solve problems of disease and delinquency we must start at the root of those problems — the diet.

In this chapter I will describe the ways we in the Cuyahoga Falls Probation Department identified metabolic problems in the people with whom we came in contact. This is not meant to serve as a handbook for professionals (those in the counseling professions may want to consult my manual, *Nutritional Guidelines For The Counselor);* it is meant to give professionals, parents and the general public an idea of how these problems are identified, and what some of their symptoms are. Granted, some of these tests are somewhat complicated and technical, requiring diagnostic equipment and trained personnel. Others, however, are based simply on careful observation and common sense. For example, I include the questionnaires we use to find out if a subject's antisocial behavior may be due to allergic reactions or hypoglycemia; professionals may use them as a guide, parents and others can use them to detect these problems in their young people. I hope this description will help de-mystify the nutritional approach, and will demonstrate the kind of simple and direct action we can take to rectify "delinquent personalities" we once believed were beyond our control.

The Reed Method

Our technique in assessing the metabolic disorders that contributed to the subjects' antisocial behavior consisted of the following steps. We began our analysis either during the presentence investigation, or as soon as the individual had been placed on probation.

1) When the person was referred to the probation department, he or she was given two questionnaires — the Schizophrenics Anonymous form and the Health Evaluator — and asked to candidly complete all three pages. We ask that the person bring the completed form with them to their first interview. The individual is not told what the questions are meant to reveal until the questionnaires are completed. Although the pro-

bationers often believe the forms are some sort of psychological inventory, they are usually quite cooperative in answering the questions completely and honestly. I think one of the most important reasons for this cooperativeness is the simple fact that we are often the first to ask these people how *they* feel.

2) On the first appointment or interview, the person was asked to write down his or her own version of what happened to cause the arrest. This account often provided information which, while it may not have been considered relevant at the trial, gave us clues as to the underlying motivations of the individual's behavior: mood swings, delusions, hallucinations, etc. It also gave me a sample for handwriting analysis, a technique I'll discuss a little later.

3) We then took a complete social history of the individual, paying careful attention to the person's health background and that of each member of the family including parents and grandparents. One of the discoveries we made is

who got in trouble with the law came from families which were plagued with diabetes, hypoglycemia, alcoholism and other metabolic disorders. Since we know that a tendency to develop such health problems can be transmitted genetically and reinforced by family eating habits and lifestyle, this observation tends to support the link between the probationers' behavior problems and their malnutrition.

4) At this point in the first interview, the counselor and the probationer carefully reviewed the probationer's responses on the questionnaires. Although the S.A. questionnaire was developed to spot warning signs of schizophrenia, I used it to detect the types of emotions and dysperceptions which were indicative of brain allergy. If the individual indicated a positive response to six or more of the 24 questions, I strongly suspected a brain allergy, or perhaps a severe nutrient deficiency or burden of toxic metals. If the person's "yes" answers fell into the 16 — 20

range, we could be certain that he or she was frequently hallucinating. In such an instance the individual was immediately referred to Baron Clinic for a complete evaluation.

The Health Evaluator questionnaire keys more directly on hypoglycemia. It is adapted from Dr. John Baron's important booklet, *Low Blood Sugar*.[4] The test is a simple tool, but it is remarkably accurate: of 5,000 persons whose response to the questionnaire indicated hypoglycemia, 96 percent were clinically confirmed to be hypoglycemic.[5]

The number of positive responses to the test's 93 questions generally falls into three ranges. If the person indicates 12 to 15 symptoms, we know that person is having significant — although not yet clinical — nutritional problems. While these problems may be having an impact on the person's behavior, and while dietary correction may bring great improvement in attitude, metabolic distortion is probably not the primary reason for their behavior problems. However, there is room here for interpretation. If the probationer indicates a positive response to any of the first five questions, complains of depression, nervousness, anxiety, tension, suicidal tendencies, waking up in a sweat, allergies or rapid pulse, or reports drinking more than three cups of coffee a day or more than the equivalent of three or four beers a day, hypoglycemia may in fact be indicated, regardless of how few other symptoms are complained of.

In absence of this, however, the subject indicating 12 - 15 symptoms is advised that he or she may be prone to hypoglycemia, and is encouraged to eliminate refined sugar and white flour from the diet.

If the subject indicates 16 - 25 of the symptoms, hypoglycemia is strongly suspected, and other nutritional problems, allergies and toxicities may also be present. In fact, a subject indicating over 20 symptoms is certainly suffering from hypoglycemia if not something more serious. Such people are placed immediately on a special whole foods diet which eliminates sugar, white flour, adrenal stimulants such as coffee or cola, and chemical flavorings, colorings and preservatives. For people with severe hypoglycemia even dairy products (which are high in milk sugar, and are at any rate highly allergenic) and high-sugar fruits like dates, figs, plums and grapes must be eliminated. The diet emphasizes fresh fruits and vegetables, whole grains, lean meats, fish and poultry, all eaten at maximum freshness with a minimum of processing and cooking. The diet is described in more detail in Chapter Four.

5) Those individuals who complain of 40, 50 or more symptoms on the Health Evaluator are suffering from severe metabolic problems. This high score often indicates sensory distortion on a massive scale, leading to a condition which is frequently diagnosed as schizophrenia. Such persons have usually already had some type of psychiatric treatment, perhaps even confinement in

a mental institution or the psychiatric ward of a hospital. Many, tragically enough, have already spent time in jail.

When possible, these people were referred to the Baron Clinic in Cleveland. Dr. John Baron is an orthomolecular psychiatrist who specializes in diagnosing metabolic disorders and treating them with a program of good nutrition, allergy prevention and detoxification. Today there are few such institutions in America, and it may be difficult for many parents or professionals in the field to obtain the kind of extensive, detailed and accurate clinical testing we have come to expect from the Baron Clinic. (The Huxley Institute can provide the name of the wholistically-oriented clinic nearest you. Its address is listed in the Appendix.)

During the subject's initial six-hour visit to the clinic, a battery of tests is performed. A six-hour Glucose Tolerance Test is usually given to reveal the exact nature of the patient's carbohydrate intolerance. Urinalysis and blood chemistry studies are performed to check sugar levels, hemoglobin counts, nutrient absorption rates, the presence of toxins, etc. A sample of the subject's hair is taken and tested for mineral and toxic metal content.

Also at this time other personality tests are made. The Hoffer Osmond Diagnostic test and the Minnesota Multiphasic Personality Inventory are often given to the patients to determine if their metabolic distortions have reached the level of schizophrenia or psychoneurosis, and, if so, what varieties of perceptual and emotional problems may be present.

6) Following the analysis of the Health Evaluator, we also did an inventory of the client's diet. I asked the probationer to recall everything he or she ate the previous day. Often this reckoning was more surprising to the probationer than to the officer; it was the first time many people made a detailed account of what they ate, and they were surprised at the amount of junk food, soda, coffee, milk or alcohol they consumed!

7) The Probation Department continued to follow up on the probationer's progress, regardless of the extent of metabolic correction required. Along with improved diet, we counseled the individual to get involved with an exercise program. The person was encouraged to spend at least 30 to 45 minutes a day walking, swimming, running, cycling, or participating in some other moderately strenuous activity. Exercise not only tones the body and improves the supply of blood to the tissues, but promotes a deeper, more restful sleep which improves a person's ability to cope with physical and emotional stress.[6] Brain researcher Dr. Richard M. Restak has concluded that "Exercise can...directly affect personality. Regular jogging and physical training can lead not only to physical fitness but also to increased emotional stability, increased imagination, and increased self-sufficiency."[7]

Obviously, a diagnostic program such as the one I have outlined above requires some major changes in the way probation officers deal with their clients. The major adaptation to be made is the realization that before behavior can be corrected, before the person can learn to control the temper tantrums, impulsiveness and poor judgment which lead to delinquent or criminal acts, the central nervous system must function properly. The probation officer, and indeed anyone who seeks to help teens or adults in trouble, must get to know as much as possible about the individual he or she is dealing with: the exact details of the person's diet, the details of the person's family life and employment, what kinds of stresses the person is exposed to. A series of rap sessions or a weekly visit from a social worker won't do the job. The counselor must, in a very real sense, become personally involved with each of the persons they deal with if he or she is going to get the kinds of results with the orthomolecular approach which my colleagues and I have accomplished.

The Diagnostic Tests

Let's discuss in detail some of the diagnostic procedures I have mentioned above. We have already examined the origin and interpretation of the S.A. Questionnaire and the Health Evaluator; it only remains for me to list them.

The Schizophrenics Anonymous Questionnaire

1) Do you feel sick all the time?
2) Are you tired all the time?
3) Are you always alone?
4) Are you shy?
5) Are you a school drop-out?
6) Did your grades drop when you reached junior high?
7) Would you rather stay inside than meet people?
8) Are you depressed, unhappy?
9) Are you afraid of heights, bridges?
10) Do you sometimes have blurred vision?
11) Do you have frequent mood

changes?
12) Do you find it difficult to concentrate?
13) Do you have trouble holding a job?
14) Do you feel that people (your family, your boss) are against you?
15) Does your family call you lazy or stupid?
16) Do you use drugs or alcohol to escape from misery?
17) Have you had thoughts of suicide?
18) Do you have a quick temper?
19) Are you fidgety or nervous?
20) Are you a chain smoker?
21) Do you have trouble sleeping?
22) Do you feel tense or depressed for no apparent reason?
23) Have you ever had a so-called "nervous breakdown?"
24) Would you prefer to separate from your friends or family rather than face reality?

The Health Evaluator

1) At times, does your mind go blank?
2) Do you become easily confused?
3) Are you forgetful?
4) Do you occasionally have difficulty with concentration?
5) Are you an underachiever in school or work?
6) Do you lose your temper easily?
7) Do you have difficulty controlling your emotions?
8) Do you have excessive sexual desires?
9) (Males) Are you impotent? (Females) Are you frigid?
10) Do you neglect cleanliness and appearance?
11) Do you have difficulty in keeping jobs?
12) Are you very impatient?
13) Do you have trouble getting along with others?
14) Do certain things irritate you very much?

15) Are you depressed, blue?
16) Have you lost interest in work?
17) Are you tired of living?
18) Are you very nervous?
19) Has your life become aimless?
20) Are you anxious and afraid but do not know why?
21) Do you have a feeling of impending danger?
22) Do you feel very tense?
23) Do you have groundless fears (phobias)?
24) Do you have crying spells?
25) Do you feel very restless?
26) Do you have suicidal tendencies?
27) Do you easily become violent?
28) Do you have a desire to cause damage to others?
29) Do you want revenge on society?
30) Does your vision suddenly become blurred or double?
31) Does sunlight hurt your eyes?
32) Do you feel dizzy or black out, especially when you stand up suddenly?
33) Do you become dizzy, stagger or

weave, especially in the morning or before meals?

34) Do you have fainting spells?
35) Are you very exhausted, especially in the morning?
36) Do you generally feel very weak and tired?
37) Are you very weak both in the morning and mid-afternoon?
38) Do you feel best after a good meal?
39) Do you feel very stuffy or sleepy after eating sweets and other starchy foods?
40) Do you feel very sleepy during the daytime?
41) Do you have trouble sleeping at night?
42) Do you wake up and cannot go back to sleep?
43) Is your sleep deep, but not refreshing?
44) Do you have cold sweats during the night?
45) Do you have no muscular strength upon awakening?
46) Do you need the stimulation of

alcohol, coffee, cigarettes or drugs? Specify which.

47) Do you feel well after eating candy, cakes or soft drinks?
48) Do alcohol, sweets and coffee make you feel very bad?
49) Do you have constipation?
50) Do you have alternating constipation and diarrhea?
51) Do you have abdominal distress?
52) Do you suffer from motion sickness?
53) Have you lost your appetite entirely?
54) Occasionally are you ravenously hungry?
55) Are you overweight?
56) Do you suffer from continuous indigestion?
57) Do you have frequent bloating?
58) Does a little alcohol make you drunk?
59) Do you crave salt?
60) Do you have terrible headaches?
61) Occasionally do you feel a pain across your left shoulder in the

direction of your collar bone or in the back of your neck?

62) Do you suffer from heat exhaustion?
63) Do you have swelling in your hands and feet?
64) Is your mouth very dry?
65) Do you have a skin disease?
66) Do your hands and legs feel cold?
67) Do you sweat excessively?
68) Is your skin dry and scaly?
69) Do you perspire very little except at the underarms, and the palms during stress?
70) Do your limbs feel numb?
71) Do you have a tingling feeling in your lips or fingers?
72) Do you sometimes wake up in a sweat at night?
73) Do you have allergies, asthma?
74) Does your heart occasionally beat very fast?
75) Do you sometimes tremble inside?
76) Do you catch colds easily?
77) Are you very susceptible to infectious diseases?

78) Do you have aching joints?
79) Do your muscles twitch occasionally?
80) Do you sometimes have cramps?
81) Do you have occasional convulsions?
82) Were you depressed after childbirth?
83) Have you had miscarriages or premature births?
84) Do you crave sweets, cakes or pastry?
85) Do you drink little water?
86) Do you drink much coffee or tea every day? About how many cups?
87) Do you drink cola and other soft drinks? About how many bottles daily?
88) Do you drink alcoholic beverages every day? How many drinks or bottles of beer do you consume daily?
89) Are you a chain smoker?
90) Are your symptoms strongest in the morning before breakfast?
91) Do you feel these symptoms gener-

ally a few hours after eating?

92) Have you had the symptoms after exhausting physical exercise or work?

93) Have your symptoms followed intensive emotional upsets?

Handwriting Analysis

As I mentioned above, I have frequently done handwriting analysis on the written descriptions taken in the first interview. Graphoanalysis, which involves the study of written strokes, can provide valuable insight into the individual's personality, helping the counselor or parent establish a better rapport. While there is no space here to describe the technique, I strongly encourage counselors to look into scientific graphoanalysis further. The address of the International Society of Graphoanalysis is given in the Appendix of this book.

The Glucose Tolerance Test

The Glucose Tolerance Test (GTT) is one of the most important tools in a program of diagnosing metabolic disorders which may contribute to antisocial behavior. After we determined from the Health Evaluator that a particular probationer might be hypoglycemic, we sent them to the Baron Clinic to find out the exact extent of the problem, and this almost always involved the administration of the GTT. It precisely maps what the body does with sugar, gives us a general picture of the entire metabolism, and provides clues to what further treatment is required.

The Glucose Tolerance Test was developed in the late 1920s as a way of diagnosing diabetes. Its basic function is to reveal a patient's blood sugar levels after the ingestion of a large amount of sugar. At that time the test was conducted for three hours; a rapid and abnormally high increase in blood sugar, which showed no significant drop by the end of the test, was considered an indication of diabetes, in which the patient is unable to produce sufficient insulin to remove glucose from the blood. But a little later in the decade, researchers like Dr. Seale Harris began to conduct the test for *six* hours, and discovered that some people showed a high blood glucose curve which was similar to that of a diabetic for the first three hours, but which ten plummeted to abnormally *low* levels. Thus hypoglycemia, or hyperinsulinism, was recognized as another type of carbohydrate intolerance.[8]

When the test is conducted, the patient is instructed to refrain from food and drink from the end of his or her evening meal until the next morning. When the patient arrives at the clinic, samples of blood and urine are taken and the content of glucose in the samples is measured. The amount of glucose in the blood, or *serum glucose*, is measured in milligrams per 100 milliliters of blood, or "mg./percent." The glucose level of this first sample is called the "fasting level." The urine should be free of sugar.

At this point the patient is given a drink which contains 100 grams of glucose, usually flavored with lemon or as a cola. Then 30 minutes later another blood and urine sample is taken, and again at 60 minutes, and at hourly intervals for the next five or six hours. The mg./percent of serum glucose is measured for each sample, and the results plotted on a graph.

There are four basic syndromes that are revealed by the GTT graph. If the person's glucose tolerance is normal, the serum glucose level will begin at a fasting level of between 80 and 120 mg./percent, and rise to a level no higher than 170 mg./percent between the 30- and 60-minute points. At about an hour, the patient's insulin production will have reached an optimum point, and as sugar is taken out of the blood, the serum glucose level will begin to drop. By the third hour the glucose level will drop to a point no lower than the fasting level, and will remain there until the end of the test. At no point should sugar be present in the urine. This is the sign of a healthy endocrine system: The body reacts in time to the abnormal ingestion of glucose, keeping the blood sugar from reaching dangerously high or low levels.

The diabetic, on the other hand, is unable to produce sufficient insulin to take glucose out of the system. In the diabetic, serum glucose rises to levels higher than 170 mg./percent in the first hour. Beyond this point, known as the "normal renal threshold," the body reacts to the glucose insult by attempting to remove sugar via the kidneys; thus glucose begins to appear in the urine (the term "diabetes mellitus" is Latin for "the sugar passes through."[9]) As the blood sugar levels continue to climb, the acid level of the blood rises, and the patient may experience weakness, dizziness, and difficulty breathing, a condition which may lead to coma.[10] For this reason, GTTs should only be conducted in medical facilities, where insulin can be administered if it turns out that the subject is in fact diabetic.

The other two syndromes are signs of hypoglycemia, in which the blood sugar eventually reaches a level at least 20 mg./percentage points *below* fasting level. Opposite of the diabetic is the patient with chronic hyperinsulinism: that is, the body constantly produces too much insulin. This is often referred to as "flat curve hypoglycemia." The blood sugar level at the fasting state may be abnormally low, perhaps around 60 mg./percent, and after glucose ingestion it may rise only 20 to 40 mg./percent points. After about an hour it begins to taper off to a point substantially below fasting level. By the end of the test it may begin to rise again slightly, may remain stable, or may continue to drop. Patients with hyperinsulinism are usually those who complain of constant hunger, tiredness or depression; their overactive pancreases never allow the blood to retain enough glucose.

The final syndrome is known as reactive hypoglycemia, or dysinsulinism. As we said in Chapter Two, it is the most common form of hypoglycemia. This syndrome is sort of a combination of diabetes and hyperinsulinism. The serum glucose level raises near or above the normal renal threshold in the first hour, and sugar may actually begin to appear in the urine. The subject's pancreas is at first unable to produce enough insulin to deal with the glucose insult. But eventually the endocrine system does react, and by the second hour serum glucose is dropping. This is where the hyperinsulin portion of the curve begins; the pancreas begins to produce *too much* insulin, and blood sugar levels plummet to below fasting levels. This blood sugar roller-coaster can be quite steep. Serum glucose may rise to 240 mg./percent, and can drop as low as to 20 mg./percent![11] It should be pointed out that this reactive hypoglycemia can be progressive. As the endocrine system deteriorates under the constant insult of refined carbohydrate consumption, the high part of the curve gets higher and longer, with the pancreas producing sufficient insulin only toward the end of the test. Such a patient is clearly pre-diabetic; soon the pancreas will cease to function entirely.

During the high portion of the curve, the patient may experience the weakness associated with diabetic acidosis, and at the low point of the curve may suffer depression, crying spells, temper tantrums or other uncontrolled emotions, or may actually black out. Even those with mild cases of hypoglycemia may suffer physical symptoms during the low blood sugar stage.

It is imperative that the patient be carefully observed during the GTT, and given something to eat to raise blood sugar again at the end of the test if there is sign of weakness or dizziness. Failure to do so can be disastrous. I know of one individual, severely hypoglycemic, who was simply sent home at the end of his GTT. In the car on the way home he went berserk, and had to be immediately hospitalized. The Glucose Tolerance Test can be uncomfortable and even dangerous if it is not given by qualified health care professionals.

It was the characteristic response of the relative hypoglycemic which helped orthomolecular psychiatrists link the disorder to psychological problems and aberrant behavior. They noticed in their patients, as I did in my probationers, that everything from sudden stupors to temper tantrums — and even murder and suicide attempts — very frequently occurred around three hours after a meal. When we began to test such individuals with the Glucose Tolerance Test, we found that the mental difficulties, physical problems, schizoid sensory distortions and antisocial behavior corresponded closely with the abnormal dips in the individual's blood sugar levels. In the area of nutrition, where so much information is tenuous and frequently in dispute, the discoveries made possible by the Glucose Tolerance Test are a very strong demonstration to the scientific community of the veracity of the orthomolecular approach.

Clinical Tests

Two of the more technical tests the clinic did for us are blood analysis and hair analysis. Scientists established the significance of such variables as nutrient and minerals levels and the presence of toxic metals to the mental health and behavior of the individual. The blood and hair tests give us some indication as to what levels of these elements are present in the subject's body.

Of course, it is easy to understand that traces of nutrients ought to be present in the patient's blood, but what of minerals and toxic metals? There was no easy way to test for the presence of these things until the advent of the hair analysis. Toxic metals and non-nutritive minerals are stored in the body's tissues. The fact that they settle in the tissues of the brain rather readily is the reason they are so damaging to a person's mental demeanor. But hair is also a tissue, and the deposits of toxic metals such as lead, arsenic, mercury, cadmium, aluminum and barium found in carefully-taken samples of the subject's hair can give us a rather precise idea of the levels of these toxins we can expect to see in the subject's body in general. If we saw a probationer whose behavior was particularly bizarre or aggressive, or whose body and physical function was deteriorating along the lines I described in the previous chapter, we immediately suspected toxic metal poisoning, and sent the subject for the necessary clinical testing.

While the hair test has proved to be a very special tool in this regard, it is not infallible. Hair analysis has an advantage over blood and urine analysis, in that, while these fluids only reveal those chemicals to which the person has recently been exposed, hair analysis reveals exposure days, weeks or months after the fact. Unlike blood samples, hair samples are easy and painless to take, and can be easily transported and stored. The test itself consists of burning the hair sample at a high temperature and then analyzing the characteristic spectrum of the light it produces for certain key elements.

But there are problems with the technique. The primary stumbling block is that medical science is as yet not sure how metals and minerals are deposited in the hair. This makes establishing a ratio of the levels of contaminants in the sample to the level in the body a very tenuous process at best. The second problem is that hair samples taken from the same head can vary in the levels of materials present, and the difference in concentration of some elements can be as much as 30-fold. In the words of Dr. Paul Lazar, Chairman of the AMA's Committee on Cutaneous Health and Cosmetics, "Present scientific knowledge does not support the use of metal levels in hair for broad, sophisticated, subtle diagnostic purposes (such as vitamin deficiencies, enzyme activity and allergic states)..."[12]

Yet the experts are not all so disparaging. Dr. Jeffrey Bland has demonstrated that, in the years since Lazar made his remarks, advancements and standardizations in hair analysis techniques have greatly improved the reliability of this diagnostic tool.[13] Dr. William Walsh, director of the Health Research Institute, has said, "I think it's only a matter of a short time before hair analysis will be accepted nationwide and worldwide. I think it's going to be a storehouse of medical information that heretofore has not been tapped."[14] I am not a doctor nor a scientist: Yet the hair analyses completed for clients have been so revealing and so consistently accurate that I cannot but agree with Dr. Walsh. While we would never consider using just hair analysis alone, I would recommend the procedure as another tool for pinpointing contributing problems.

We often use a clinical testing service in Illinois, Doctor's Data, Inc., which not only does very accurate testing but also sends us the findings in the form of a page of computer-generated line graphs which give us a vivid picture of what is happening with the subject's biochemical makeup. Dr. Oscar Rasmussen, a biochemist in Chicago highly skilled in hair analysis interpretation, has assisted since 1976. There is also a numerical value given for the level of an element found in the individual, and a normal numerical range given with which to compare the subject's levels.

The two-sheet prognosis report lists and graphs the subject's levels of calcium, magnesium, sodium, potassium, copper, zinc, iron, manganese, chromium, cobalt, lithium, molybdenum, nickel, phosphorus, selenium, silicon, and one or two others which may be present in the individual system. Levels of toxic metals listed above are also given numerically and graphed.

An important and often overlooked fact is that nutrients seldom work alone. As we saw in Chapter Two, the biochemical reactions which make them useful to the body usually only occur in the presence of other nutrients, making the body's biomolecular processes a vastly intricate and highly interconnected system. Our clinical testing service takes this into account, and includes in the report data pertaining to the ratio of minerals in the subject's body which must be balanced in order to function. We are given the ratio of calcium to magnesium, zinc, phosphorus and manganese; the ratio of copper to zinc and iron; the ratio of cadmium to copper and zinc; and the ratios of magnesium to potassium, sodium to potassium, potassium to zinc, iron to manganese, lead to calcium, and mercury to selenium.

Also included in the printout are a general explanation of the findings, a description of the sources of nutrients and toxins and their effect on the body, and a list of suggestions on how to increase nutrient levels, or eliminate toxic materials.

Despite the detail of such testing, it is relatively inexpensive. Again I must stress that medical science has not yet established any absolute link between the hair content of these elements and their concentration in the body. But we find that it is very helpful to have this information, especially for probationers who display chronic or severe problems which a simple change to a whole foods diet isn't likely to immediately remedy. We must know what is happening with the body's metabolism before we can begin to correct it.

For a graphic example of how important such clinical testing is, let us look at the test results for Raymond, the young man who was brought before me for attempting to murder his girlfriend and whose case I described in detail in the introductory chapter. We'll go through Raymond's report in the same way I review the findings of all the patients we send for clinical testing.

The first variable we check is the toxic metal levels, and in Raymond's case these were quite dramatic. For instance, the maximum level of lead which is acceptable in the human body is 15 parts per million: Raymond's hair sample contained more than 32 parts per million. As I explained in the previous chapter, lead interferes with cellular enzymatic reactions which leads to such problems as lack of energy, listlessness and gastrointestinal discomfort; all of these were symptoms of which Raymond complained. His hair sample also showed 1.26 parts per million of cadmium, over 25 percent in excess of the maximum the body can handle. High cadmium levels decrease the body's ability to absorb and use nutrients, an effect which was exacerbating all of Raymond's other metabolic difficulties. He also showed levels of arsenic, mercury and barium which approached the maximum acceptable limits.

As it turned out, we easily traced the source of Raymond's toxic metal contamination: His heavy inhalation of gunpowder fumes, when he practiced his marksmanship, contributed to it. It is not, however, always a simple task to trace the source of toxic metal intake. The storage and effects of these poisons are cumulative, and the body has no way of quickly eliminating them. We often find that our probationers are suffering from the effects of a toxic metal contamination that occurred years before they got into trouble with the law. High levels of metallic toxins are usually treated by dietary therapy, often in combination with the process of chelation. I will explain these therapies in more detail in the next chapter.

The next findings we examine are the levels of nutrient minerals, especially copper, zinc, iron, manganese and chromium. Exceptionally low levels of a particular nutrient tell us either that the subject is not getting sufficient amounts of the nutrient in his or her diet, or that some metabolic difficulty is preventing his or her body from absorbing the proper levels of nutrients from the food he or she consumes. Exceptionally high levels suggest overconsumption of a food rich in those nutrients, or a nutritional deficit elsewhere which is preventing the body from using the minerals.

Raymond had problems in both areas. His level of sodium was 366 parts per million, compared to the normal range of 22 to 163 parts per million. Likewise, his potassium levels were at 178 parts per million, compared to the normal rate for his sex and age of 11 to 80 parts per million. The overabundance of these nutrients was directly attributable to Raymond's junk food diet — junk and processed foods are excessively high in salts, and people who live on them are commonly getting as much as 25 times the amount of salt they need. Raymond's excessive levels of these nutrients were contributing to his feelings of anxiety and his inability to concentrate and apply himself to a task.

On the other side of the coin, Raymond's test results showed a marked deficiency in several vital nutrient minerals. His tests revealed a magnesium content of 23 parts per million, compared to the minimum normal range of 32 to 122 parts per million. Magnesium is vital to the metabolism of sugar, salt and vitamins — it was apparent that Raymond's high carbohydrate diet was probably responsible for his magnesium deficiency. This in turn contributed to the feelings of mental disorientation and confusion and the hair-trigger temper with which Raymond was beset.

He also had dangerously low levels of calcium (25 percent deficient) and copper (10 percent deficient). These deficiencies probably also contributed to his mental lassitude and aggressiveness. Raymond's mineral ratio chart pointed out that it was indeed his overconsumption of sodium and potassium, as well as the massive amounts of toxic metals in his system which caused the calcium and magnesium deficiencies. Raymond's problems in these areas were eventually corrected through the use of chelation and dietary therapy.

From this thumbnail description, it is easy to see that clinical blood and hair testing is vital to an orthomolecular approach to solving psychological and behavioral problems. As I have said above, such testing can sometimes be difficult to obtain. Right now there are only 15 hair analysis laboratories in the nation.[15] Such a factor may dissuade probation departments and other professionals from using the tests, especially when they have never been required to do diagnostic testing of any sort in the past. But I hope this case study demonstrates how useful such testing is in pinpointing the exact biochemical stresses which influence each individual case of delinquent behavior. I am certain that if more professionals in my own discipline and all those who deal with delinquent teens and adults, were to start making more use of the biochemical testing services already in existence, there would be a growth and expansion of such facilities. The cost would also be reduced.

This, then, is the method we use for determining the metabolic problems which we have come to see as some of the root causes of delinquent behavior in the probationers I have dealt with. In the next chapter, I will explain in detail the dietary regimen on which we placed our clients, as well as some of the clinical therapies on which we rely in cases of more extreme metabolic distortion. I feel that, although this orthomolecular approach to the problem of delinquency, criminality and mental illness requires a much more thorough relationship between counselor and subject, psychiatrist and patient, parent and child, it is not overly expensive or difficult to implement. And the results are well worth the effort.

NOTES

[1]D.J. Kallen, "Nutrition and Society," *Journal of the American Medical Association,* 1971, Vol. 215 No. 1, p. 94.

[2]Carl C. Pfeiffer, *Mental and Elemental Nutrients,* (New Canaan, Connecticut: Keats Publishing, 1975), p. 3.

[3]Medard Gabel, with the World Game Laboratory, *Ho-Ping: Food for Everyone,* (Garden City, New York: Anchor Press, 1979), p. 28.

[4]John Baron, *Low Blood Sugar,* (Cleveland, Ohio: Karpat Publishing Company, Inc., 1971).

[5]Nola A. Smith, *Investigation of Hypoglycemia as a Causal Factor in Some Kinds of Emotional Distress,* (Unpublished thesis, Eastern Michigan University).

[6]Thomas Kirk Cureton, *The Physiological Effects of Exercise Programs on Adults,* (Springfield, Illinois: Charles C. Thomas Publisher, 1971).

[7]Richard Restak, *The Brain: The Last Frontier,* (Garden City, New York: Doubleday and Company, Inc., 1979), p. 76.

[8]E.M. Abrahamson and A.W. Pezet, *Body, Mind and Sugar,* (New York: Avon Books, 1977), pp. 53-54.

[9]"Diabetes," in William Morris, ed., *The American Heritage Dictionary of the English Language,* (Boston: Htughton Mifflin Company, 1978), p. 363.

[10]"Diabetes," in *Dorland's Medical Dictionary,* Shorter Edition (Philadelphia: The Saunders Press, 1980), p. 199.

[11]The foregoing discussion of GTT curve interpretation adapted from Abrahamson and Pezet, *Body, Mind and Sugar,* p. 55.

[12]Laura A. Engleman, "Unlocking Your Medical Profile: The Inside Story on Hair," *Vegetarian Times,* Sept. 1982, p. 24.

[13]Jeffrey Bland, *Hair Tissue Mineral Analysis,* (Bellevue, Washington: Bellevue Redmond Medical Laboratories, Inc., 1979).

[14]Engleman, "Unlocking Your Medical Profile...," p. 23.

[15]Engleman, "Unlocking Your Medical Profile...," p. 25.

CHAPTER FOUR

HEALING THE DELINQUENT MIND: THE ORTHOMOLECULAR APPROACH

The doctor of the future will give no medicine, but will interest his patients in the care of the human frame, in diet, and in the cause and prevention of disease.
— Thomas A. Edison

No illness which can be treated by diet should be treated in any other manner.
— Maimonides[1]

What are we to do about crime and delinquency? Must offenders be written off as social and moral basket cases, kept as captive wards of the state for the rest of their pitiful lives? Can anything be done to *prevent* crime, short of caging or killing human beings in the name of deterrence?

While most Americans are beginning to view the growing crime rate as a hopeless problem, the dreariest outlook is held by those charged with seeing justice done, those within the criminal justice system itself. Listen to criminologist Alexander Schauss:

> Currently, the criminal justice system is going nowhere. Instead of spending money to seek effective rehabilitation for criminals and prevention of crime, the money is being spent on larger and more secure institutions and jails. Habitual offenders are viewed as hopeless. Each such declaration costs the taxpayer from $7,000 to $25,000 a year. With over 300,000 prisoners in United States correctional institutions, this is a substantial drain on the American economy. Additionally, each year over one million children are detained for some period of time in juvenile detention centers across the country. It costs from $6 to $35 a day to hold a child in one of these facilities.[2]

Clearly, we are spending huge amounts to cope with our crime and delinquency problem. But where is it getting us? In the decade between 1968 and 1977, a time when expenditures on law enforcement programs, courts, prisons and rehabilitation programs climbed to record figures, the number of murders rose 38.6 percent. Forcible rape nearly doubled. Aggravated assault climbed 82.2 percent, and robbery was up 54 percent. All together, crimes of violence increased nearly 70 percent during the period.[3]

An interesting study appeared in the *American Psychologist* in 1978, a study that's not talked about much in psychiatric circles. The study reviewed the lives of 500 participants in the famous Cambridge-Somerville Youth Study of 1939. The boys had been chosen as "difficult" or average by officials from schools, welfare agencies, churches and police departments. They were given physical examinations and interviewed, and then were rated according to the likelihood that they would become delinquent.

The boys were then put in matched pairs according to age, delinquency proneness, family background and home environment. One half of each pair was randomly placed in a treatment program for five years. The other boy received no treatment at all. One third of the boys in the treatment group received family-centered therapies; over half got a special tutoring in academic subjects; over 100 received medical or psychiatric attention; a quarter were sent to summer camp; and most were put in contact with Boy Scouts, YMCA and other community programs. In short, for five years the boys in the treatment group got the best that medicine and psychiatry could offer in the way of delinquency prevention; the boys in the non-treatment group got nothing.

Thirty years later, Joan McCord of Drexel University examined the life histories of these men as revealed by hospital files, court records and other documents. What she discovered should have shaken the criminal justice, psychiatric and medical professions to their very foundations — if anyone had paid attention. She found that:

1) Men who had been in the treatment group were *more* likely to commit at least one more crime if they committed a first

than those who got no treatment.

2) Men who had been in the treatment group were *more* likely to show signs of alcoholism.

3) Men who were in the treatment group were *more* likely to show signs of serious psychiatric illness.

4) Men from the treatment group died younger.

5) Men who had been in the treatment group were *more* likely to report having had at least one stress-related disease, especially hypertension and heart disease.

6) Men from the treatment group were *more* likely to have a lower-prestige job, and to find that job unsatisfying.

In sum, McCord's study showed that the magic programs that social workers, psychiatrists and welfare agents swore by as delinquency prevention methods were *worse* than useless; *they actually did more harm than good!*[4]

We rely on the police, courts and prisons to bring offenders to justice and to keep them "off the streets" until and unless they are no longer a danger to society. Yet the criminal justice system seems little more than a hopeless, lethargic merry-go-round, on which the same individuals spin for a lifetime in an endless cycle of arrest-release, arrest-release. According to FBI statistics, out of a sample of 207,748 persons arrested from 1970 to 1974, 65 percent had been arrested at least twice before. Among the ten most frequent repeat offenses were murder, rape, assault and weapons crimes. Another study, this one released in 1972, found that 67 percent were re-arrested within three years.[5]

All the while, the courts and prisons are increasingly flooded with cases, and those rehabilitation programs that exist are woefully unable to keep up. To an increasing extent our correctional facilities are merely warehouses in which criminals pace out their sentences, growing ever more bitter, ever more isolated from a society in which they are unable to function, ever more adept in the ways of crime.

According to a growing number of researchers, this is all they will ever be. The more moderate conclude that "In seeking to make criminal justice more redemptive and less punitive, we may have asked too much of institutions that can barely hold their own, let alone develop the competence to be curers of souls..."[6] Others are more blunt: "Wicked people exist," says James Q. Wilson. "Nothing avails except to set them apart from innocent people."[77]

In the case of the worst offenders, public reason turns to public rage. More states are reviving the death penalty, and the ranks of those waiting to die at the hands of the state are swelling. Executions have become media events, the condemned is made a household word, and shots of the pleading parents and the outraged citizenry dominate the evening news. It seems that centuries of social development have brought us at last only a very little way from the headsman and the chopping block.

In this era of pervasive hopelessness

about crime and delinquency, can there be any alternatives, any untried paths, which can possibly lead us out of this dark labyrinth of violence and fear?

I believe there is such a path. It is a path along which I myself have traveled, along with thousands of probationers. Every one who has stayed on the path has reached daylight, has never been in legal trouble again. Today they live normal, healthy, happy lives. And the first step down this path is the realization that *a healthy body means a healthy mind.*

We must recognize that crimes are not committed by "criminal minds" or even "antisocial personalities;" they are committed by whole persons. While the quality of an individual's upbringing and the environment in which a person lives are doubtlessly important, we must begin to recognize that one's physical state, and particularly the molecular environment of the brain, plays a crucial role in shaping behavior. Schauss puts the biochemical connection in precise proportion:

> The contributing factors to juvenile delinquency are many. For decades, the problem of juvenile delinquency has been seen as the product of only social and intrapsychic factors. Families have been seen as the cause of delinquency. Criminologists have largely ignored disturbed biochemical functioning as a possible cause of criminal behavior. It is just such an interest in our biochemical environment, as achieved by a study of diet and delinquency which is needed to redress the balance.[8]

No one is suggesting that we ignore the psychic and social components of crime and delinquency. I *am* saying that we ought to spend at least as much effort in healing the body as we have in "curing the soul."

The path I'm talking about is called the *Orthomolecular Approach* — "ortho" from the Greek for correct, and "molecular" from molecule. Orthomolecular treatment simply means providing, in Linus Pauling's words, "the right molecules in the right amounts."[9]

Although the orthomolecular approach to the treatment of mental and behavioral disorders is sometimes pictured as unorthodox or even "flaky" by establishment physicians embarrassed at their own failures, the approach is in fact based on two very sound concepts. As we saw in Chapter Two, brain function is actually a set of thousands of complex chemical processes, each of which requires the presence of the proper molecules in order to work properly. If these molecules are not present, or if some other substance (such as a toxic metal) is preventing the molecules from taking their proper places, then the brain malfunctions, and behavior is distorted. It follows, then, that if we are faced with an individual who behaves abnormally, we ought to determine first if there are any chemical distortions in the brain, and, if there are, we ought to correct these imbalances. Certainly other influences of behavior — the individual's ability to deal with others, conflicts which may stem from his or her upbringing, etc. — should be dealt with as well. But there can be little reason to expect that such procedures alone will be of much value when the brain of the subject is malfunctioning.

This, then, is the foundation of the orthomolecular approach: *the restoration of the proper molecular balance of the brain.* The primary tool for this restoration is diet; however, vitamins, minerals and other food supplements may also be used, as well as certain drugs which help to remove toxic materials from the body. The orthomolecular technique is almost never used alone, but as an adjunct to counseling and other types of therapy.

What sort of molecular balance *is* proper for the brain? Or, put another way, what is optimal brain nutrition?

It would be foolish to attempt to give a complete answer to a question like this. In the first place, despite the smug confidence of the government bureaus who set MDAs and RDAs, science simply doesn't know terribly much about nutrition. We don't even really know how many nutrients there *are*. As of this writing, nutritional science has isolated 45 nutrients, all of them thought to be essential to human health. Just 30 years ago, the list was perhaps half that. No one knows how many new nutrients may be discovered in the future; we *do* know, however, that when we try to build chemically complete mock-ups of certain foods, they do not support animal life as well as the natural foods themselves.[10]

We do not fully understand even those nutrients we have managed to isolate. In 1973 the USDA asked several nutrition specialists for their opinion as to the current state of our knowledge of nutrition. The scientists were questioned about 46 specific nutrients, and asked to state whether substantial progress had been made in our understanding of the nutrient, whether only fragmentary data had been collected, or whether data was poor or nonexistent. The nutritional needs of different age groups were considered. In the area of adolescent nutrition, the scientists said that *no substantial progress had been made.* Partial data existed for ten nutrients, and only poor or non-existent information was available for 36 nutrients. For young adults, nutritional knowledge was only a little clearer: substantial progress had been made for 16 nutrients and fragmentary data had been collected for another 10, but little or no data existed for 20.[11] Clearly biochemists and nutritionists are not prepared to make any definitive statements about human nutrition.

A more fundamental reason we can't make any hard-and-fast statements about human nature stems from the concept of biochemical individuality. As we saw in Chapter Two, and as the work of Dr. Roger Williams has demonstrated,[12] each individual organism is unique, and each has its own nutritional requirements. Two women who are the same age and weight can have significantly different needs; one may require only 500 mg. of vitamin C a day to maintain good health, while the other may need 1,500 mg. or more. It will do little good to refer to a chart in order to prescribe a proper diet for two such women, even though they may be "identical" as far as the USDA is concerned.

What I am saying here is that, in the field of nutrition, it is useless and often counterproductive to rely on some figure which is claimed to represent someone's "average" dietary needs. There are no average people, and in determining proper brain nutrition one has to be careful to concentrate on the specific needs and responses of each individual.

Given all of this, is there anything we can say in general about proper brain nutrition? There is. In the first place, *proper brain function requires the presence of all essential nutrients.* This seems a bit obvious at first, perhaps, but it's a point which is frequently overlooked in most discussions of nutrition. Each chemical process in the body involves the interaction of scores of nutrients, and the function of these often depends on the presence of scores of others. In fact, Doctors Harte and Chow have established that the absence of a single nutrient can create a metabolic "shock wave" which hinders the function of all the rest.[13]

This simple fact takes on new importance when we remember that food processing robs foods of a broad range of vitamins, minerals and enzymes, while "food enrichment" puts back only a few. No enriched food that I know of contains added zinc or choline, for instance, although both of these are removed in processing. Very frequently the food industry argues that, because the action of many micronutrients is not yet fully understood, we don't have to worry about them.[14] This sort of reasoning is extremely odd; most vitamins, for instance, were first noticed because animals or humans deprived of them become ill. Just because we don't yet know precisely what zinc does in the body doesn't mean we can ignore the fact that people with zinc deficiencies suffer nervous system disorders. To say that we ought to pay no attention to the less "popular" nutrients simply because scientists don't know all about them is a little like arguing that since I don't know the chemical difference between gasoline and diesel fuel, it makes no difference what I put in my car. Your body knows what to do with the nutrients it needs — and that's all that really matters.

From what we said about the nutritional damage done by food processing, it follows that the best way to get the full range of essential nutrients is to eat unprocessed foods — whole, fresh, natural foods. Natural foods are foods for which the processing has been kept to an absolute minimum; they have been left raw or are only lightly cooked, and all edible skins, seeds, bran and germ remain. Such foods contain virtually all their original nutrient value because they have not been subjected to milling, boiling, flaking, puffing, extruding, and other nutrient-destroying processes. It should be added that whole, fresh foods not only contain a good supply of the vitamins, minerals and enzymes that we know about; evidence suggests that such foods also contain nutrients we have yet to discover.[15]

Another general requirement of proper brain nutrition is that *most carbohydrates should be complex carbohydrates from high-fiber foods, and simple sugars should be kept to a minimum.* The complex carbohydrates are the starches, found in whole grains, potatoes, squash and many kinds of vegetables. The starches, like sugars, provide energy for the body. Unlike sugars, however, unrefined carbohydrates break down much more slowly into glucose — and consequently don't contribute to severe fluctuations of the glucose level affecting brain functions.

It is important that carbohydrate foods be eaten with plenty of fiber. As we pointed out in Chapter Two, fiber is a plant substance which does not break down in the stomach. It helps to move digested food smoothly through the intestine, and moderates the absorption of carbohydrates. Even starchy foods can break down too quickly into glucose and cause a hypoglycemic reaction, if fiber is completely absent.

Once again, the best source of complex carbohydrates and fiber is whole, natural food. Those nutrient-rich parts of food which are thrown away during food processing — the skins, seeds and bran — are also the richest sources of fiber. So while a meal of stripped, deep-fried potatoes may distort the body's metabolism, a baked potato eaten with the skin provides just the energy-food the body needs.

Protein should be derived from lean meats and vegetable sources. We have already noted that, while the adolescent needs a good supply of protein, this protein is very often obtained from beef (hamburger is the big offender), which is high in fat and not very well digested. Optimally, one's protein ought to come from meats like chicken (not fried), fish and veal, which have higher protein-to-fat ratios and are easier to digest — I like to refer to them as the "gentle proteins." Also, vegetable protein sources (nuts, beans, peas, lentils, whole grains) ought to be more widely consumed. Although few single vegetable protein sources are as "complete" as meat, mixing two of them (like brown rice and beans) provides an excellent range of amino acids, as well as fiber and other nutrients lacking in meat.[16]

Fats ought to be kept to no more than 10 percent of total caloric intake. While a moderate intake of fatty acids is very important in human nutrition, too much fat can be damaging. The metabolism of fat creates ketones, substances which are hard on the kidneys and other organs. Also, as we said before, high fat consumption leads to increased levels of serum cholesterol, and cholesterol deposits can block blood flow to the brain.

When I criticize the amount of fat the average American eats, I am indirectly attacking the major contributor of fat to our diet — fast foods. The rise in American fat consumption — from about 35 grams per person per day in 1920 to 70 grams in 1976[17] — has closely paralleled the growth of the fast food industry, with its vast store of french fries, onion rings, hamburgers, fried chicken, and "thick shakes" (thick because the milk has been replaced with hydrogenated vegetable fat). The USDA has admitted that the increased popularity of convenience and snack foods, as well as hamburger joints and carry-out chicken and fish restaurants, have contributed greatly to our herculean intake of fat.[18]

Fresh unprocessed foods, on the other hand, are quite low in fat — with the exception of nuts and seeds, which ought to be eaten in moderation (the high-fiber content of these foods helps insure they *will* be eaten sparingly).

When an oil is desired for cooking or for a salad dressing, I recommend the cold pressed oils — olive oil, safflower oil, sunflower oil and a few others. These are called "cold pressed" because they are extracted from foods with a high natural oil content, and so require less heat in processing than corn oil or seed oils do. In addition, compressors and other equipment are kept cool. The lower heat preserves the essential fatty acids intact, while these nutrients may be destroyed in the processing of other kinds oils. (Once opened, cold pressed oils must be refrigerated to prevent rancidity.)

For bread-spreads or baked potatoes, butter is better. Yes, butter contains animal fat and margarine doesn't, but the human body is set up to digest small amounts of animal fat. Margarine is a completely synthetic product, made of hydrogenated vegetable fats, chemical stabilizers and artificial flavors. I like biochemist Paul Stitt's assessment of margarine: "The taste may say 'butter,' but the ingredients say junk."[19]

Fresh, whole fruits and vegetables, lean digestible meats, natural cold-pressed oils — these are what a person ought to eat in order to get the best possible nutrition for the brain. By the same token, you ought to avoid white flour, white sugar and other kinds of refined carbohydrates, fatty meats and fried foods, adrenal stimulants like caffeine and nicotine, and artificial colors, flavors, preservatives, emulsifiers, stabilizers and additives of all kinds. Naturally, you should also avoid any foods to which you are allergic.

How can you find the foods that best nourish the brain, and avoid those foods which cause mental malfunction? My favorite strategy is to shop around the perimeter of the supermarket. That's where all the fresh produce is! When you come to the meat and dairy cases, you'll have to be a bit cautious. Pass by the beef and processed meats, and remember that all those things that look like cheese and butter may be the concoction of some profit-mad scientist. As much as possible, avoid the center of the store, with its aisles of canned, boxed, bagged, over-sugared, nutrient-stripped, low-fiber, high-chemical monstrosities. If you want to pick up a box of tissue or a six-pack of mineral water, you may go in — but hurry right back out!

Although this plan for surviving the supermarket is helpful, it is even better to shop at co-ops which offer organic produce — fruits and vegetables which have been grown without the use of chemical fertilizers, pesticides or herbicides. I recommend organic produce because it contains fewer trace poisons than traditionally-grown food (although in our chemically-inundated ecosphere, it's impossible to avoid these poisons entirely). The chemical traces in regular produce can set up an allergic reaction in some people,[20] and they're really no good for anyone.

In addition, it's easier to tell if organic produce is fresh. Most commercial produce is waxed, dyed and sprayed to retain the appearance of freshness, so that it can be stockpiled and warehoused for months and still look just-picked. This warehousing greatly reduces the vitamin content of produce; biochemist Robert J. Benowicz maintains that "These warehouse impostors are a kind of subtle junk food that delivers 'empty' calories as surely as the processed kind."[21] Organic produce is not doctored this way, so that if it looks fresh, it *is* fresh; if it's not, it looks old and moldy, just as over-ripe produce ought to. And since you buy them fresh, organic fruits and vegetables are much more nutritious than the supermarket kind.

Thirdly, organic farmers are careful to maintain the nutrient content of the soil, so that produce is more nutritious. Regular farming techniques, however, deplete the soil, so that the fruits and vegetables raised on it don't reach their nutritional potential.[22]

The watchword throughout this discussion of brain nutrition has been "natural." The best way to get the best nutrition is to eat natural foods, foods which are fresh and whole and as unprocessed as possible. Now, I'm certainly not the first person to make this prescription; the natural foods movement has been growing for decades. The result is that an increasing number of shoppers are on the lookout for natural foods, and more food manufacturers are attempting to convince consumers that their products are natural. In fact, "100% Natural" is quickly replacing "New and Improved" as the most over-used phrase in the American supermarket.

Some people (especially food industry flacks) have hailed this change as an example of the food giants bending to consumer demand for healthier food. Yet this "natural revolution" is fraught with charlatanism. Many so-called "natural" foods have been canned, freeze-dried, flaked and puffed — hardly the sort of things that go on in the wilderness. For instance, a lot of foods billed as natural, especially natural snacks, contain brown sugar. Brown sugar is thought to be more natural than sucrose, probably because it's brown. In fact, brown sugar is simply white sugar with a little molasses or brown food coloring added, and it can lead to hypoglycemia every bit as much as its lighter cousin. Some producers of "natural foods" don't even bother with this bit of sleight-of-hand,

and simply add sugar or corn syrup to their products, because these at least haven't come straight from a test tube!

White flour — often called "wheat flour" to confuse the unwary — is another frequent ingredient in misnamed "natural" foods. Many "whole wheat" breads, for instance, actually contain little whole wheat flour. When shopping for a whole grain bread, look for a good firm loaf. Bread calling itself "whole wheat" which is soft and squishy is usually made up of white flour, dough conditioners and brown food coloring. A recent Consumer's Union study showed that such phony "wheat breads" are just as nutritionally barren as white breads.[23]

The point is that just because a product may say "all natural" on the package, just because it may be brown or contain coconut, doesn't mean it's really a whole, natural food. *Read the label.* If it lists any of the offending ingredients we've talked about, or contains anything that even appears to be a chemical additive, don't buy it. Moreover, it's best to avoid anything in a can or a box; nature doesn't put food in cans or boxes. Some food industry spokesman might reply, "Nature doesn't put food in supermarkets, either, which is absolutely correct. Nature puts food in gardens and farms, which is where you ideally ought to get most of what you eat. Start a garden, if you can; shop at farmers' markets and road-side stands whenever possible.

Let's look at how these nutritional principles translate into a specific dietary program.

THE REED DIET

I use this diet to help correct the metabolic imbalances of my probationers. As I mentioned in the last chapter, if a person complains of 15 or more symptoms on the hypoglycemia questionnaire, he or she is placed on this correctional diet. And it is a *correctional* diet, designed for people in pretty poor health. As a result, it is a bit more strict (especially in the area of high-sugar fruits) than a diet made to help *prevent* behavioral problems.

ALLOWED FOODS

PROTEIN: All lean meats (beef, pork, lamb), chicken, fish, turkey, eggs, cheese, yogurt, legumes, nuts.

WHOLE GRAINS cooked or soaked: Cracked wheat, rolled barley, steel-cut or rolled oats (not quick), brown or wild rice, whole millet, etc.

VEGETABLES, fresh or frozen (to be eaten raw or lightly steamed):

Artichoke, asparagus, avocado, beet greens, black-eyed peas, broccoli, brussels sprouts, cabbage, cauliflower, carrots, celery, collards, corn, cucumbers, eggplant, garlic, kale, lentils, lettuce, lima beans, mustard greens, mushrooms, okra, onions, peas, peppers, pumpkin, pumpkin seeds, radishes, sauerkraut, soy beans, spinach, squash, string beans, sunflower seeds, swiss chard, tomatoes, turnips, turnip greens, watercress, and homemade vegetable soup.

In the diet I use, it's open season on fresh, raw vegetables; we urge probationers to eat plenty every day.

FRUITS, fresh or frozen: Apples, apricots, berries, cherries, fresh coconut, grapefruit, kumquats, lemons, limes, mango, melon, papaya, peaches, pears, pineapple, tangerines. (It is permissible to eat fruit with a little cream — if you're not allergic to milk, of course — but no sugar may be added.)

JUICES, fresh or frozen: Apple, cranapple, grapefruit, orange, pineapple, tomato, vegetable, Vegemato, V-8.

BEVERAGES: Spring or distilled water (6 to 8 glasses daily, addition of *fresh* lemon or lime optional), any of the above mentioned fruit juices (in moderate amounts), buttermilk, milk (in moderation, again if there's no allergy), herb tea, Fresca (if you *must* have a soft drink, drink this in moderation), vichy water, sparkling mineral water, kefir, carob soda — no sweeteners.

SNACKS: Raw sunflower seeds, raw pumpkin seeds, popcorn (little or no salt and butter), banana chips, granola, hard-boiled eggs, blueberries, cantaloupe, avocado, dried pineapple rings, sprouts (sunflower, alfalfa, soy, mung), cottage cheese, cheese slices, cold roast beef, cold chicken, yogurt (plain or with added *fresh* blueberries, nuts or other fruits — beware of commercial

yogurts with sugared fruit flavorings), nut mixes (with raw nuts).

Additional notes: As stated above, only cold-pressed oils should be used for cooking or salad dressing (with a little apple cider vinegar).

Eat only whole-grain bread and baked products (wheat, soy, rye, corn, oatmeal, etc.) with no preservatives.

When you think about it, the *allowed foods* list covers a vast range. In fact, it represents more dietary variety than most people in our society ever enjoy. Certainly no one on this diet need feel deprived! There are, however, some substances which have no place in this diet:

STRICTLY FORBIDDEN FOODS

Avoid *all* refined sugar and flour, or products made with them (the only way to be sure of this is to read labels carefully).

Avoid foods with artificial additives, coloring, preservatives or sweeteners.

Do not consume bakery products such as pastries, cake, pie, or other desserts such as puddings, Jello, chocolate.

Avoid coffee and coffee substitutes such as Sanka and Decaf (Cafix and other grain-based coffee substitutes can be purchased in health food stores), Coca Cola, Pepsi and other pop, diet or otherwise. Instead, drink the listed fruit juices, herb teas, or — surprise! — water.

Avoid grapes, prunes, dates, raisins and figs. (We suggest hypoglycemics do this for at least four to six months, as these fruits contain a great deal of natural sugar.)

Avoid pre-packaged, instant foods.

Avoid all refined starch foods, such as macaroni, spaghetti, rice, noodles (except soy noodles), potatoes, ravioli, pizza. (Many of these products are now made with whole-grain flours, and these are perfectly acceptable.)

Avoid all medications containing caffeine.

Avoid beer, cocktails, cordials, wines.

It ought to be added that, in case of extreme addiction to some of these substances (sugar and caffeine in particular), we do not try to take probationers off "cold turkey" — the withdrawal symptoms are simply too extreme. Instead, we urge them to cut back. For instance, if an individual is addicted to coffee, we suggest they first switch to decaffeinated coffee (which still contains some caffeine), and then attempt to give it up altogether. In the same way, if a person is consuming many bottles of soda a day, we will try to help them replace some of the soda with fruit juice, while at the same time urging them to drink several glasses of water a day. This way thirst for sugared soft drinks is diminished as gradually and naturally as possible.

Some people swear by the "cold turkey" approach,[24] but I feel that some of my probationers would become so violently ill if suddenly taken off caffeine or sugar that they would not stick to the diet.

Any good diet has two parts, of course: it contains a list of foods, and it prescribes a way of eating. In our diet, probationers are given a carefully planned eating schedule designed to provide the right nutrients at the right time, and to maintain stable blood sugar levels:

EATING PATTERN

Upon arising — drink (slowly) 8 oz. of water and 4 oz. vegetable, fruit or tomato juice (this gets the digestive juices flowing, and makes a person hungry for breakfast).

Breakfast (within 20 minutes of juice) — high protein foods such as eggs and whole grains (see list). A slice of whole-grain bread or toast, fresh fruit or melon and a cup of herb tea would be one menu for a nutritious breakfast. You might also want to try a bowl of homemade

soup, brown rice with broiled fish, melted natural cheese on whole wheat bread, etc.

One hour after breakfast — glass of water.

Mid-morning snack (two hours later) — selection from snack list (raw sunflower and/or pumpkin seeds are recommended here).

One hour after mid-morning snack — glass of water.

Lunch — high protein foods (see list) with a raw vegetable salad, slice of whole grain bread.

One hour after lunch — glass of water.

Mid-afternoon snack — yogurt, buttermilk or vegetable juice.

One hour after snack — glass of water.

Dinner — should include protein, with plenty of lightly cooked vegetables and/or a raw vegetable salad. Fresh fruit for dessert.

One hour after dinner — glass of water.

Light evening snacks (every two hours until bedtime — selection from snack list).

You'll notice a lot of snacking is permitted — even *required* — on this diet. This is because a hypoglycemic's haywire carbohydrate metabolism needs constant propping up. Frequent snacking will help maintain blood sugar levels, and fight off those light-headed, dizzy or shaky feelings hypoglycemics suffer a couple of hours after eating. We often recommend that people carry a snack mixture with them, so that if they're ever caught away from home, they aren't without nourishment.

The proper breakfast is crucial. The body needs plenty of high-quality protein at the beginning of the day to prepare itself for the action and stress to come. So for those who don't have time to fix a more elaborate breakfast, I recommend this fast, high-protein drink:

Put 5-6 ounces of unsweetened juice (cranapple, apple, pineapple, orange or grapefruit juice will do) in a blender and set it on low.

Add 2 tablespoons prepared protein (powder or liquid),

1 teaspoon Brewers yeast (gradually increase this to 2 teaspoons over a period of four weeks, if not allergic to yeast),

1 teaspoon cold-pressed safflower oil,

1 teaspoon raw honey (optional),

1 tablespoon millers bran (if you have a problem with constipation).

Other optional ingredients — ½ ripe banana and raw egg yolk.

Set blender to high and blend for 30 seconds. Drink slowly.

The combination of ingredients in this breakfast drink may sound a little unusual, but give it a try. Even fitness fan Richard Simmons was surprised by how good it tastes when I first introduced it to him.

We encourage people to add as much variety as possible to their diet, with the goal of eating no single food twice within four days. We have found that this four day cycle helps the body remove allergy-producing substances. The technique is particularly effective for those persons with allergies to many different foods. For specific rotation diets (which can sometimes be quite complex), consult Philpott and Kalita's excellent book, *Brain Allergies,*[25] or Dr. Marshall Mandel's book, *5-day Allergy Relief System* (See Appendix).

After the proper diet has been established, we begin to explore the probationer's need for vitamins, minerals and other food supplements. Supplements will not be effective in the absence of a well-balanced diet. The variety of micronutrients needed to help metabolic processes can only be gotten from food. Food supplements can help replace lost nutrients or make up for unusual needs, but they cannot replace a good diet. The point may seem a little simple, but many people today think they can compensate for a diet of the most horrifying junk simply by taking a multi-vitamin at breakfast. Indeed, the pharmaceutical companies which push such supplements encourage this view in their advertising. It's okay if your kids subsist on potato chips and soda all day; just pop a One-A-Day in their mouths and things will be all right. Nothing could be further from the truth.

Once we've established a proper diet, however, we can begin to assess a person's need for added supplementation. Frequently a probationer's supplement regimen will look something like this:

B-Complex vitamins, 50 milligrams — 1 or 2 at every meal (the breakfast drink I described provides a good supply of B vitamins, so supplementation may not be needed at this meal).

Vitamin C, 500 milligrams — 1 or 2 at each meal. The body uses up more vitamin C in times of stress, and few people are under more stress than a juvenile or adult in trouble with the law. It is important that the daily intake — some 1,500-3,000 milligrams — be taken in small doses throughout the day, rather than in one large tablet at breakfast, since the body tends to wash out any vitamin C it can't immediately use. If you take a lot of vitamin C over a long period of time, *never* suddenly stop taking it. The body becomes accustomed to a regular supply of vitamin C, and sudden discontinuation may cause scurvy-like symptoms. At no time should the supplementation of vitamin C fall below 500 milligrams daily, although certain individuals (especially alcoholics and other chemical abusers) may benefit from doses much higher than 3,000 milligrams.

Vitamin A, 10,000 units — 1 or 2 daily. This dosage should normally not be exceeded. Vitamin A is one of the few nutrients which, in excessive amounts, can cause toxicity. Because it is fat soluble, it stays in the body's fat tissues rather than washing out readily. Prolonged overdosage (more than 100,000 units daily for adults) can lead to hair loss, nausea, vomiting, diarrhea, skin problems, fatigue, headaches and liver enlargement.

These warnings aside, however, it

must be noted that vitamin A is one of the most frequently missing nutrients in processed foods, and supplementation in order to correct long-standing deficiencies is frequently required.

Vitamin E, 200 to 400 International Units — 1 with each meal. Another fat-soluble nutrient, vitamin E is frequently removed from grain in the milling process, because the volatile oils in which it is found shorten shelf life. Those who have been trying to subsist on white flour products often need supplementation of this nutrient.

Multi-mineral supplement — take as directed. As we saw in Chapter Two, many minerals are very important for proper brain function. In addition, keeping levels of beneficial minerals high helps prevent toxic metals (especially lead) from taking the place of nutrients in brain processes.

Papaya Enzymes — Take as directed. Many probationers complain of indigestion, and anybody knows what chronic indigestion can do to a person's emotional state. The enzymes found in papaya help break down nutrients in the stomach and digestive tract, and prevent indigestion.

Chromium — When an individual is an alcoholic, we frequently recommend chromium supplements to reduce the craving for alcohol.

L-Glutamine, 500 mg. with each meal — Glutamine has been found very effective in helping to reduce the craving for sweets, alcohol or drugs. L-Glutamine is a substance that is often referred to as the "memory pill," as it also helps improve memory.

This, then, is our diet. It is an emergency program for people whose metabolisms have become so imbalanced that their behavior gets them in trouble. If the probationer sticks to this program, we expect to see a definite improvement in his or her health and outlook within four to six days, although in many cases complete recovery may take weeks or months.

This is an important point to note. The

orthomolecular approach is a means of helping the body recover its natural equilibrium; it is not an interventionist technique; it does not interfere with any other physical systems in order to get some short-term psychiatric benefit. It is not a quick fix. Many people are so used to the rapid effects of mood-altering drugs which are frequently prescribed for persons with behavior problems that they wonder why it may take several days or even weeks before an improvement is seen. This is why it must be remembered that the orthomolecular path seeks to *heal* the individual, to *correct* the imbalance, rather than simply cover up unwanted behavior.

The diet I outline in this chapter is correctional. Some of the foods on the forbidden list may be eaten in moderation once the body has been restored to health. However, we do recommend that if people are especially sensitive to one of the forbidden foods (or even foods on the allowed list, although these are normally hypo-allergenic) that they omit this food from their diet permanently.

Getting people to try the Reed Diet is not always easy. The offenders I saw often had severe addictions to some of the very foods that were killing them. They usually lack self-discipline, and, since the court had ordered them to see me, they very often resented anything I tried to tell them, to say nothing of the radical changes I asked them to make in the way they ate.

Some of them never stick to the diet, and these are the ones who usually get back into trouble with the law. Some change their diets for awhile, until a personal crisis forces them back into their old eating habits. More frequently, a probationer will try the diet for about a week, figure there's nothing to it, and give up. But the orthomolecular diet has a built-in hook for such people: normally, when an individual goes off the diet after four to six days, their former mental, behavioral and physical problems return so fast that it's obvious even to them. They no longer need me to convince them they need a correctional diet — they have witnessed the proof in their own bodies. They become true believers.

There's one last facet of this orthomolecular program which I must mention again: EXERCISE. We encourage probationers to engage in at least 30 to 45 minutes of strenuous, rhythmic activity — jogging, biking, swimming, jazzercise, even walking — every day or a minimum of four times a week. Exercise not only tones up the entire body and builds up the ability to deal with stress; it also increases the blood and oxygen supply to the brain, and studies show it can vastly improve mental health.[26]

The Orthomolecular Approach And Other Therapies

I feel that the orthomolecular approach to healing mental and behavioral problems has several distinct advantages over the kinds of treatments normally offered in such cases:

1) *It is safe.* We expect safety from all healing techniques; after all, one of the rules of the Hippocratic Oath is "First, do no harm." But the fact is that one of the most frequent types of treatment for behavioral disorders — the prescription of tranquilizers and other mood-altering chemicals — can be quite dangerous. It's not unusual for some of my probationers to be arrested under the influence of one or more prescription psychoactive drugs, and much of the mental confusion they experience can be linked to these drugs.

A tranquilizer never cures depression, anxiety or other emotional disorders. It only slows down the central nervous system. At the same time, it can do quite a bit of damage. One common substance prescribed for psychiatric patients is chlorpromazine, packaged by Smith Kline & French as Thorazine. According to the *Physician's Desk Reference,* Thorazine is indicated for the management of psychotic behavioral problems, for severe or violent hyperactivity in children, to control nausea and vomiting and to relieve restlessness and apprehension in patients before surgery. The FDA has classified Thorazine as *possibly* effective for control of excessive anxiety, tension and agitation as seen in neuroses.

One thing is certain: Thorazine can have a number of harmful side-effects. Their listing takes up more than two and one-half columns in the PDR! They include drowsiness, jaundice, blood disorders, infection, low blood pressure, neuromuscular reactions resembling Parkinson's disease, uncontrollable rhythmic motions of the face and mouth (which may be irreversible in some patients), psychotic and catatonic-like symptoms, convulsive seizures, allergic reactions, discoloration of the skin and visual impairment. There have even been cases of sudden death as the result of cardiac arrest after administration of the drug, although no one is yet sure if the heart attacks were actually caused by Thorazine.[27]

Granted, these dangerous side-effects associated with Thorazine and other psychoactive drugs do not occur all the time in all patients — but anyone who takes them is at risk. And when you remember that many patients are taking two, three or more of these drugs simultaneously, you begin to appreciate the risk involved.

The orthomolecular approach, on the other hand, is completely safe. It interferes with no other physical systems in order to heal the mind; in fact, it enhances the health of the entire body. I have recommended dietary correction to thousands of probationers, and my colleagues have used orthomolecular treatment in thousands of additional cases. I have yet to hear of a *single* serious health complication which has resulted from such an approach. How many psychiatrists who rely on psychoactive drugs, electroconvulsive therapy or lobotomy can make a similar claim?

2) *It is inexpensive.* Recall the figures that Alex Schauss cited at the beginning of this chapter: juvenile detainees cost the taxpayer as much as $35 a day, and

prison inmates cost up to $25,000 a year. For those whose violent, irrational behavior makes hospitalization or institutionalization necessary, the costs to their families — or to the taxpayer — are even heavier. Yet it seems that, under current methods of treatment and rehabilitation, costs only increase, while positive results are hard to find.

Because nutritional therapy is so simple, it is very inexpensive. For example, the staff at one home for delinquent boys found that when they replaced sugar and processed food with fresh, whole food, their food bills actually decreased![28] While clinical tests for metabolic disorders and required food supplements are an added expense, their cost is always much lower than that of drugs and lengthy hospital stays. Best of all, patients who get orthomolecular treatment often shorten their probation periods or prison sentences, find jobs and live productive lives — rather than remaining as economic burdens to their families or to the state.

3) *It works.* More and more institutions which deal with delinquent or criminal individuals have been using dietary correction as an adjunct to their regular programs. The results have been very encouraging, especially to those who had lost faith in the very notion of rehabilitation. There are so many success stories that it's hard to know where to begin to describe them. But I think it's best for me to start closest to home — with my own experience with the orthomolecular approach.

Success Stories

I am completely convinced that dietary therapy is one of the most powerful tools available for the treatment of emotional and behavioral disorders. Certainly, it is not the only tool; counseling and other rehabilitative techniques are also valuable. But we must remember that a person with a sick brain is fundamentally unable to participate fully in the counseling process, or to take full advantage of rehabilitation programs. Probationers who are overcoming their health problems, however, are much more responsive to other types of treatment. More than 80 percent of the probationers who have come to me since I started using the orthomolecular approach are living full, productive lives today. *Not a single individual who has stuck with the program has ever been in trouble with the law again.* This success has been so convincing that many professionals at the Municipal Court of Cuyahoga Falls have simply taken it for granted. The connection between diet and crime, and the effectiveness of the orthomolecular approach in restoring self-control to people with behavioral problems, is accepted as a simple fact.

Let me tell you the stories of some teenagers who were thought to be hopeless, people who had lost control of themselves, people on the verge of despair — yet people who are now rebuilding their lives. I could fill volumes with statistics, but to me the most convincing evidence in support of dietary therapy lies in the success stories of people like these:

R.S. — This 19-year-old man had been receiving psychiatric treatment since his mid-teens, and at the time of his arrest for indecent exposure he was on seven different psychoactive medications. He masturbated constantly in front of others, and suffered severe headaches, night sweats, depression and inability to concentrate. His mother had spent thousands of dollars trying to help R.S., and had flown him all over the country to consult respected psychiatrists, but to little avail. His condition only seemed to get worse.

As is routine, we asked R.S. to fill out our hypoglycemia questionnaire. We were shocked at what we found — 58 symptoms of hypoglycemia! We sent him to the Baron Clinic, where he was indeed diagnosed as hypoglycemic. But that wasn't all. A hair analysis indicated his system was loaded with lead, and his liver was malfunctioning. R.S. was one of the worst cases of metabolic distortion we had seen; little wonder his behavior was so bizarre.

We placed R.S. on a nutritional program to correct hypoglycemia and gave him treatments to remove the toxic metal from his body. His recovery was dramatic. Within weeks his family noticed a marked improvement in his behavior and attitude. Six months later he took the hypoglycemia questionnaire again, and this time he showed only eight symptoms. The numbers spoke for themselves. I recently telephoned R.S.'s mother, and she assured me he was doing fine — healthy, happy and out of trouble.

D.L. — This 18-year-old was referred to the probation department after he had been caught shoplifting. His was a rather typical case. D.L. ate as most adolescents in this society eat — he consumed a lot of fast-food lunches and plenty of snack foods and cola. It was no surprise when he indicated over 30 symptoms of hypoglycemia. We urged him to give up refined carbohydrates and adopt the diet mentioned in this chapter. D.L. also got involved in jogging as a part of his exercise program.

D.L. has not been in trouble again since adopting the diet. And he stuck with the exercise; today he is a promising marathon runner.

M.K. — This young man was 19 years old when he was convicted of driving under the influence of alcohol and possessing marijuana. His alcoholism had reached such an advanced stage by the time of his arrest that he was committed to an alcohol/drug treatment program for nearly a month. When his time there ended, his probation began, and that's when I saw him.

M.K.'s alcoholism was being fueled by hypoglycemia, as evidenced by the fact that he craved and consumed enormous amount of refined sugar, caffeine (from colas and coffee), candy, donuts, etc. when not drinking alcohol.

We attempted to correct M.K.'s hypoglycemia, and combined this with megadoses of certain vitamins. He got two grams of vitamin C a day in four 500 mg. doses, as well as two grams of nicotinamide (a form of niacin) and L-Glutamine, and a multiple vitamin and mineral supplement.

M.K.'s progress would have heartened all those who have despaired of successfully treating alcoholism. Within three weeks he was jogging up to five miles a week, and in four months he was running five miles a *day*. He said he felt like a new person. His self-esteem improved wonderfully, and in the five years since then he has never returned to drugs or alcohol, and has not been in trouble with the courts.

S.B. — Fourteen-year-old S.B. had had a tough life. He was considered a poor learner; he got D's and F's in everything, and required special education programs. Behaviorally S.B. was a problem as well. He had already been arrested three times for burglary and theft. Even though he had been through child guidance, juvenile court and intensive psychological therapy, nothing had helped. His father was referred to my office — the boy was helped as a result.

When S.B. was given a Glucose Tolerance Test at the Baron Clinic, it was discovered he was severely hypoglycemic. His diet bore this out — he survived on ice cream, pop, donuts and candy. We worked with his parents to help turn his diet around.

Once again, the results were swift. Within two grading periods he was able to enter regular classes again, and got on better with friends and schoolwork. He got a part-time job, and his grades improved to B's and C's. Today he's graduated from high school, has a full-time job and plays in his own band. He has not been in trouble since beginning the corrective diet.

As remarkable as this change was, S.B. said it took him three years before he was completely convinced that it was sugar that was responsible for his problems. But looking back, he realized, "Whenever I ate sugar I got so bad my friends didn't want to be around me." Yet today, the boy that the teachers and psychologists had given up on is a bright and alert young man.

I should point out that the orthomolecular approach works with people over 20 as well:

N.S. — This 51-year-old woman was referred to me after she was convicted of petty theft. Her life had been a catalog of emotional crises; for the last several years she had grown continually more tense, argumentative and confused. Physicians had placed Mrs. S. on powerful tranquilizers, and these contributed still further to her inability to cope with life. She had been hospitalized eight times for tranquilizer overdose, and for months had been unable to drive or work.

When Mrs. S. and her husband first came into my office, I had to recheck my files to be sure I had her age right. This woman didn't look 51 years old; I could swear by the way she tottered in on her husband's arm, peering dimly around, that she could have been 80. She was depressed, exhausted, couldn't keep her balance, and had been losing her vision. She could scarcely pay attention during our interview.

Privately, her husband told me of his desperation. He could no longer tolerate life with this woman who was swiftly becoming a physical and emotional cripple. "As soon as she gets a little better," he said, "I'm divorcing her."

As the two of them left my office, N.S. clung to her husband for support. When they got to the door, the man let go of his wife for a moment to search for his car keys. She toppled over, coming to rest in a crumpled heap against the wall.

I knew this woman was a victim of something more than mere emotional stress. I sent her to the Baron Clinic for a glucose tolerance test. My suspicions were confirmed: N.S. was hypoglycemic.

Immediately Mrs. S. was placed on the corrective diet I described earlier. Her recovery was almost immediate. After only one week of treatment for low blood sugar, she was once again able to drive a car. In two weeks she returned to work. When she made her routine appearance in court two and one-half months later, she was clearly a changed woman. Once again I doubted her official age; this time she looked *younger* than 51! She was bright, alert, energetic. She told the judge she hadn't felt so good in 10 years — and no one challenged her testimony.

To this day, N.S. has been out of trouble. For a probation officer, that is gratification enough. But there's another happy sidelight to this success story: as Mrs. S. regained her mental and physical health, her husband, who had been so ready to end their marriage, fell in love with her again. As she returned to her former self, her husband followed her around like a teenage sweetheart. For N.S., orthomolecular treatment saved a marriage — and salvaged a life.

D.D. — D.D. was a pretty, dark-haired

30-year-old who was brought to me after her arrest for driving under the influence of drugs. But D.D. was no patron of back-alley dope dealers; the drugs which got her into trouble were prescribed.

D.D. had a history of emotional instability. For eight years she spent much of her time in a psychiatric ward. In 1968 she became terribly depressed over the death of her dog, and her doctors responded by putting her on seven different psychoactive drugs. In addition, in the four years from 1968 to 1972 she received over 50 electroshock treatments.

Her world was a waking nightmare. She frequently felt that she was floating in space, looking helplessly down at her own inert body. She would black out for long periods. There were days when she would simply lie in bed, struggling to maintain her tenacious grip on reality. "That is my dresser," she would tell herself. "It really is my dresser. I am lying in bed. I am really here."

Her doctors voiced concern over the quantities of drugs she was taking.

"You've really got to control your drug use," they told her, but they continued to provide a steady supply of mood-altering chemicals. At last they attempted to take her off drugs entirely, but her withdrawal symptoms were severe: she shook constantly, and could not rally the strength even to go to the bathroom. Admitting failure, the doctors put her back on "medication." She was under the mind-bending influence of these drugs when she was arrested.

When I first saw D.D., she was a mess. Her eyes were dull, her hair looked dry and brittle, and she seemed depressed, exhausted and tense. I asked her to fill out the standard hypoglycemia questionnaire, and she indicated 42 symptoms. Dr. Baron's diagnosis confirming hypoglycemia came as no surprise.

Corrective therapy was not an easy experience for D.D. She found the diet inconvenient at first, and she could hardly choke down the vitamins which were prescribed to help correct her nutritional imbalances. But she gave the program her grudging tolerance; "I'll stay on the diet long enough to get off probation," she told herself. "Then I'll do what I want."

Things didn't work out the way D.D. had planned. After a year on the program her physical and mental health improved so remarkably that she didn't *want* to return to drug abuse. Today D.D. is in glowing good health, and is living a normal, drug-free life. Her long nightmare is over.

L.R. — I did not meet L.R. until he was 31, but like so many of my probationers his problems started in adolescence. He had been in trouble with the police since the age of 15.

He had been put on probation after being charged with telephone harassment. Getting a menacing phone call from L.R. must have been a chilling experience. His voice was hollow and lifeless, as if it were coming from somewhere far away. He told me his body felt dead — and I could easily believe it. He *looked* dead.

L.R. had a number of physical and emotional problems which were ruining his life. He suffered excruciating headaches and frequently broke into drenching sweats. His alcoholism was growing worse. Despite his 130 I.Q., he had lost several jobs, and was on the verge of losing the one he now held. L.R. had seen psychiatrists for four years before his arrest, but they had helped little.

L.R. indicated 49 symptoms on the written hypoglycemia test, and was placed on a corrective diet. He seemed to come alive before our eyes. Within a week the sweating and headaches had stopped. By the end of 1976 his appearance and behavior had been transformed, and he got a promotion on the very job he had been in danger of losing. But the "new" L.R. was not content merely to hang on — he wanted to move up. He went back to school to study civil engineering, and married a legal secretary. L.R. is once again a living man.

These recoveries may seem miraculous, but at the Municipal Court of Cuyahoga Falls they are a regular occurrence. I have seen hundreds of other probationers every bit as desperate as these make full recoveries. And for every hopeless case like the ones above, there have been thousands of simple shoplifters, drunk drivers and street brawlers whose lives have been similarly reclaimed through nutritional therapy. I have seen it happen far too many times to dismiss it as coincidence or fluke or as the result of some "placebo effect." The orthomolecular approach *works*.

And I am not alone in my enthusiasm for dietary correction. Hundreds of institutions have tried the technique and are sold on it. There is simply no room here to list them all, but let me mention some that have attracted the most attention.

The most recent and exciting verification of the nutritional path came in a 1980 study of kids in a juvenile detention home on the East Coast. The behavior of the boys who ate this home's "normal" menu (high in sugar and processed foods) was compared to that of a later group of boys whose sugar intake was secretly reduced. Of course, the dietary changes themselves were noticeable: Sugar syrup was washed off canned fruit, fruit juices replaced sugared soft drinks, honey replaced table sugar, and high-sugar breakfast cereals, jelly and sugared cinnamon were removed. But neither the boys nor the staff of the home were told that the aim of the menu changes was to reduce sugar intake, or that the boys' behavior was being studied.

The results were astonishing. The 24 boys on the reduced-sugar diet showed a 45 percent lower incidence of formal disciplinary actions than the boys on the earlier diet. A separate group of eight boys who had been incarcerated before the diet change was studied as a "before and after" group. They showed a 55 percent reduction in disciplinary actions after sugar was reduced in their diet, a drop which is far too large to be attributed to "learning the ropes" at the home.[29]

Alex Schauss has demonstrated in a controlled study the value of the nutritional approach as a tool for probation officers. A study sample of 102 misdemeanant probationers was divided into four groups. One group received nutritional counseling, one group was shown nutrition education material, and the other two groups got conventional casework and counseling. Probationers given nutritional information were significantly less likely to be re-arrested than those who got standard counseling. In fact, the combined recidivism rate of the nutrition groups was 14.7 percent, less than half that of the control group.[30]

Dr. Carolyn Brown is Executive Director of The Growing Mind, an institution in Berkeley, California, which provides orthomolecular treatment for violent and delinquent juveniles. Early health problems convinced her of the link between hypoglycemia, allergies, toxicities and behavior. In Congressional testimony in

1977, she told of her enthusiasm for the nutritional approach:

> We have seen incredible results in the last two years. The most noticeable one is the one related to blood sugar. If we give these children protein every two hours, their behavior is kept very much in better control. Compared to that first two or three months, the difference is amazing. The children are learning to read, depending on their disabilities. The children have truly moved ahead. They probably would have been the kind of children that would never have been in school again.[31]

Another remarkable person, Tamara Youngman, runs a small group home for young people with behavioral problems in Fairmount, Illinois. The home is called the Purple Heart Homestead. Youths at the homestead are put on a vegetarian diet. In addition they are given dietary drug detoxification, as well as vitamin therapy to correct any metabolic distortions caused by past drug abuse. The orthomolecular treatment that juveniles get at the Purple Heart

Homestead has proven effective in eliminating their mood swings and aggressive behavior. Youngman and the Homestead have developed a reputation throughout the state for rehabilitating youths who had been kicked out of other programs, written off as hopeless.[32]

The dietary approach has also proved effective in other areas of criminal justice. Officials at the Montgomery County Detention Center in Maryland have found that inmates were unruly and had poor morale when continually served pre-packaged, processed meals. Their behavior improved when they were given a diet containing less sugar, more fresh fruits and vegetables, and whole grain bread.[33] Chief Warrant Officer Gene Baker of the U.S. Naval Correctional Center in Seattle, Washington has seen similar improvement in detainees when refined carbohydrates were removed from the diet and replaced with whole foods. Baker began the program in 1978, and a year later was able to write:

> Since this time, the medical log

> shows a definite decrease in the number of confinees at sick call and on medication has occurred, and that disciplinary reports for this year are down 12 percent from the same time frame of last year.[34]

Nor is this all. The orthomolecular approach has also been found helpful in controlling hyperactivity in children,[35] and alcoholism,[36] schizophrenia[37] and neuroses[38] in juveniles and adults.

With the repeated successes of nutritional methods, one would think that orthomolecular treatment would be revolutionizing our criminal justice system. Unfortunately, it is not. Ignoring scientific evidence and thousands of clinical reports, many in the psychiatric, law enforcement and rehabilitation communities still dismiss dietary treatment as quackery. The orthomolecular approach isn't "high-tech" enough; it isn't complicated and expensive; it doesn't require powerful drugs and armies of M.D.'s — how could it possibly be effective? Alex Schauss, one of the handful of experts in the field of diet and behavior, sums up the scope of ignorance concerning the orthomolecular path:

> When I spoke before both the National Juvenile Court and Family Judges Association and the California Legislature's Commission on Crime Control and Violence Prevention, members of both groups expressed a concern that criminal justice officials and schools were ill-equipped to diagnose or treat children and youths who have biochemical imbalances and break the law. They are correct. Through 1981 virtually no training of criminal justice officials exists in any English-speaking country that draws upon the wealth of medical and scientific information potentially of practical value of such officials.[39]

America has yet to reap the enormous potential for saving lives — and saving billions of dollars — offered by the orthomolecular approach. But I believe that it is an idea whose time has come, an idea with an intrinsic power which will overcome all remaining barriers. When it does, it will have a tremendous impact on every aspect of the criminal justice system, from parent to prison guard. It is the vast implications of the orthomolecular approach to which we now turn.

NOTES

[1]Moses Maimonides, quoted in William Philpott and Dwight Kalita, *Brain Allergies,* (New Canaan, Connecticut: Keats Publishing Inc., 1980), p. 3.

[2]Alexander Schauss, *Diet, Crime and Delinquency,* (Berkeley, California: Parker House, 1981), p. 95.

[3]Theodore B. Dolmatch, ed., *1980 Information Please Almanac,* (New York: Simon and Schuster, 1979), p. 818.

[4]Joan McCord, "A Thirty-Year Follow-Up of Treatment Effects," *American Psychologist,* March 1978, pp. 284-289.

[5]Leonard Broom and Philip Selznick, *Sociology: A Text With Adapted Readings,* Sixth ed. (New York: Harper and Row Publishers, 1977), p. 427.

[6]Philip Selznick, "Preface" in Elliot Studt, Sheldon L. Messinger and Thomas P. Wilson, *C-Unit: Search for Community in Prison,* (New York: Russel Sage, 1968).

[7]James Q. Wilson, *Thinking About Crime,* (New York: Basic Books, 1975), p. 209.

[8]Schauss, *Diet, Crime and Delinquency,* p. 3.

[9]Linus Pauling, "Orthomolecular Psychiatry," in David Hawkins and Linus Pauling, eds., *Orthomolecular Psychiatry,* (San Francisco: W.H. Freeman and Company, 1973), p. 2.

[10]Scott Knickelbine, "Boy oh Boy, Do We Have Plans for You: The Food Industry," *Acres, U.S.A.,* September 1982, p. 9.

[11]Information from the Nutrition Institute, Agricultural Research Service, United States Department of Agriculture, quoted in "Supplementation of Foods vs. Nutrition Education," *Food Technology,* July 1974, p. 58.

[12]Roger J. Williams, *Biochemical Individuality,* (Austin, Texas: University of Texas Press, 1977).

[13]R.A. Harte and B. Chow, "Dietary Interrelationships," in M.G. Wohl and R.S. Goodhard, *Modern Nutrition in Health and Disease,* 3rd. ed. (Philadelphia: Lea and Febiger, 1964), pp. 534-544.

[14]Tom Gorman, "Now We Know — Wheat Does Beat White..." *Bakery,* June 1981, p. 53.

[15]Knickelbine, "Boy oh Boy...", op. cit.

[16]Frances Moore Lappe, *Diet for a Small Planet,* (New York: Ballantine, 1975).

[17]Michael F. Jacobson, *The Changing American Diet,* (Center for Science in the Public Interest).

[18]Select Committee on Nutrition and Human Needs, United States Senate, *Dietary Goals for the United States,* (Washington: U.S. Govt. Printing Office, 1971).

[19]Paul Stitt, with Mark Knickelbine and Scott Knickelbine, *Fighting The Food Giants,* (Manitowoc, Wisconsin: Natural Press, 1980), p.74.

[20]Philpott and Kalita, *Brain Allergies,* p. 156.

[21]Robert J. Benowicz, "The Age of Vitamins," *Family Health,* September 1980, p. 30.

[22]Joe D. Nichols and James Presley, *"Please, Doctor, Do Something"* (Old Greenwich, Connecticut: The Devin-Adair Company, 1972), p. 25.

[23]"Breads", *Consumer Reports,* September 1982, pp. 438-443.

[24]William Dufty, *Sugar Blues,* (New York: Warner Books, 1975), p. 206.

[25]Philpott and Kalita, *Brain Allergies,* pp. 28-49.

[26]Richard M. Restak, *The Brain: The Last Frontier,* (Garden City, New York: Doubleday and Company, Inc., 1979), p. 76.

[27]"Thorazine," in Charles E. Baker, Jr., ed., *1981 Physicians' Desk Reference,* (Oradell, New Jersey: Medical Economics Company, 1981) p. 1691.

[28]Stephen J. Schoenthaler, "The Effect of Sugar on the Treatment and Control of Antisocial Behavior," *The International Journal for Biosocial Research,* 1981, Vol. 3 No. 1, pp. 1-9.

[29]Ibid.

[30]Alexander G. Schauss, "Differential Outcomes among Probationers Comparing Orthomolecular Approaches to Conventional Casework/Counseling," *Journal of Orthomolecular Psychiatry,* 1979, Vol. 8 No. 3, pp. 158-168.

[31]Testimony of Dr. Carolyn Brown, in Select Committee on Nutrition and Human Needs, United States Senate, *Diet Related to Killer Diseases, V: Nutrition and Mental Health,* (Washington: U.S. Govt. Printing Office, 1977), pp. 44-54.

[32]Schauss, *Diet, Crime and Delinquency,* pp. 6-7.

[33]Select Committee on Nutrition, *Dietary Goals, p. 52.*

[34]*Schauss, Diet, Crime and Delinquency,* p. 6.

[35]Ben F. Feingold, "Dietary Management of Behavior and Learning Disabilities," in Sanford A. Miller, *Nutrition and Behavior,* (Philadelphia: Franklin Institute Press, 1981), pp. 235-246.

[36]E. Cheraskin and W.M. Ringsdorf Jr., with Arline Brecher, *Psychodietetics,* (New York: Bantam Books, 1974), pp. 43-56.

[37]David Hawkins, "Orthomolecular Psychiatry: Treatment of Schizophrenia," in Hawkins and Pauling, *Orthomolecular Psychiatry,* pp. 631-673.

[38]Kay Hill, "Orthomolecular Therapy Review of the Literature," in Roger J. Williams and Dwight K. Kalita, eds., *A Physician's Handbook on Orthomolecular Medicine,* (New York: Pergamon Press, 1977), pp. 184-195.

[39]Schauss, *Diet, Crime and Delinquency,* p. 15.

CHAPTER FIVE
IMPLICATIONS

I believe that the most important pathway to mental and physical health is the conviction that improvement is possible, no matter what the condition or the age of the person may be.

— Lendon Smith[1]

The paradigm that is replacing (old medical views of human sickness) is, of course, orthomolecular medicine because it...gather(s), like butterflies in a net, all the bits and pieces of widely diversified research and crystaliz(es) them into a new image of man.

— Helen G. First[2]

I am always surprised that so many of my colleagues are surprised that nutrition has something to do with behavior.

— Abram Hoffer[3]

In this book we have examined in much detail the connection between food and behavior. We have looked at the ways diet can influence the subtle chemistry of the brain, seen some of the techniques used to determine if a behavior problem has a metabolic root, explored a diet which has proven enormously effective in helping to correct behavior, and looked at the great triumphs of the orthomolecular approach. With the force of current research and clinical experience firmly behind the concept that proper nutrition can prevent delinquency and crime, we too may be a little surprised that anyone still doubts the links between nutrition and behavior.

But the fact is that we live in a society whose hospitals, schools, universities, courts, prisons and mental institutions are formed around models of human behavior far different from the ones offered by the orthomolecular psychiatrist. I and others believe that the failure of these institutions to cure, educate, readjust and correct is traceable to the failures of these underlying models. Furthermore, we feel certain that the adoption of the orthomolecular model will require society to re-think the ways that these institutions are run.

The orthomolecular approach to mental and behavioral problems is revolutionary yet the revolution it proposes need not be a bloody one. To the contrary, our experience has been that nutritional and orthomolecular approaches are tremendously liberating concepts. The orthomolecular nutritionist, far from replacing the parent, teacher, psychologist, judge or social worker, helps all of these to carry out their roles in a much more effective and successful way. And there's nothing more gratifying than success.

What precisely are the implications of the orthomolecular approach for those who deal with juvenile delinquency and other kinds of behavior problems?

Parents

Nutrition begins at home. Parents are responsible for far more than just what their kids have for supper; the food-behavior habits they instill almost from the moment of birth will influence how the child will think about food for the rest of his or her life. If the child is allowed or even encouraged by the example of his or her parents to indulge in processed foods, junk foods, refined sugar, cola or coffee, cigarettes or alcohol, then that child will continue those habits after leaving home, and will in all probability join the swelling ranks of the victims of heart disease, diabetes, hypoglycemia, cancer, psychosis and schizophrenia which clog our nation's hospitals and prisons. If, on the other hand, the child is taught to value and enjoy whole, fresh fruits and vegetables and learns to associate what he or she eats to how he or she feels, then that child will almost certainly grow up to be a healthy, happy, fully functioning adult. This is not to say that your kids will never have problems in life; they will, however, have the biological equipment necessary to deal with problems in healthy and constructive ways.

I have heard a common complaint from parents at the hundreds of seminars I have given across the United States: "My kids just won't eat decent food!" One of the rationalizations often used to justify the processed and sweetened fare served in the school cafeteria is that children just won't eat anything else. Sometimes this line of reasoning is taken to absurd lengths.

I remember one woman who begged me desperately for some way to get her child off junk foods. "She just stuffs herself with candy and other garbage all day long," the mother told me. "How can I stop her?"

"How old is your daughter?" I asked.

"Three years old."

If the situation weren't so dreadfully serious, I might have laughed aloud. Surely no three-year-old is able to make the capital outlay for a day's supply of junk food (to say nothing of being able to reach the checkout counter). Our children cannot become "sugarholics" without our cooperation. If you don't buy this poisonous stuff for your kids, they won't be able to eat it.

If your children are already in their teens, of course, the task of reforming their diet is more difficult. More of their food decisions are made outside the home, where supervision is impossible. Peer pressure can have a great impact on the nature of these decisions — and those who turn down cola, candy, pizza and alcohol may be ostracized as "weird." At home, the sugar-addicted teen may be a bit more forceful than the pre-schooler in resisting any change in his or her diet.

And, whether the child in question is a tot or teen, any dietary change must take place in a *family* context. Getting rid of the Coke in the refrigerator and the cake on the table will affect all your children, as well as a wife or husband who may be far from convinced that any change is needed. (Getting the whole family exercising eases and aids the transition.)

Needless to say, no sure-fire method exists for "de-junking" your family. But the two watchwords for any such effort are *education* and *moderation*. Let your family know how the things they eat can make them feel. This book can help in that regard; I have listed other excellent resources in the Appendix. Have them watch for their *own* reactions to food. You can lecture someone about hypoglycemia all you want; it's when they feel that weakness, hunger and irritability two hours after a meal that they really begin to catch on.

Moderation is also important. It's probably never a good idea to run through the kitchen, throwing away all the breakfast cereal and chocolate milk. The three-year-old will scream; the 13-year-old will revolt. I've found it best to systematically "forget" to buy those processed and junk foods that your children crave. Forget the macaroni and cheese one week, the popsicles the next, the white bread the next. At the same time you can be replacing these unhealthy food items with fresh fruits and vegetables, whole grain breads and cereals, lean unprocessed meats and cheeses and nuts.

While you are the major influence on your child's eating behavior, you are unfortunately not the only one. Television — especially the programming aimed at children — is filled with commercials proclaiming how delicious, desirable and wholesome all those chips, candy bars, cakes and soft drinks are. The Food and Drug Administration and the Federal Communications Commission refuse to limit or regulate these attempts by multinational conglomerates to seduce our children into eating things that can do them no good, and a great deal of harm. The television networks simply run a couple of 30-second cheap puppet shows about the importance of vegetables and claim they've done their best at "self-regulation."

While we certainly ought to protest these massively-funded attempts on the lives of our children, we as parents must take direct action if we are to protect kids from this kind of exploitation. Finding things for kids to do as an alternative to watching TV is a good first step, although demanding that they *never* watch is probably a bit too stringent. Try not to use the television as a babysitter, however; watch TV *with* your kids, and help them understand that something is not good to eat just because the clown on the screen says it is. One sharp mother I know makes a game of this: "What's *this* commercial trying to make us think?" she asks, and her kids are getting pretty good at ferreting out the misinformation being pushed on the tube.

Another source of influence on your child's eating behavior is school. What we learned in the elementary school classroom is, for too many of us, all we may ever know about nutrition. Even today, the quality of nutrition education in our schools gives us little reason for optimism. A 1982 review by the Center for Science in the Public Interest showed that four of the five major high school health textbooks completely ignore the important Dietary Goals issued by the

U.S. Senate Select Committee on Nutrition and Human Needs, that three of them make little mention of dangerous food additives, and most contain only poor to average discussions of the dangers of too much salt, fat and cholesterol, while understressing the need for dietary fiber.[4] It is not unusual for the "educational material" distributed in many classrooms to be free hand-outs from major food companies.

The damage done in the classroom is often compounded in the cafeteria. Here the student is confronted with meals which, while they may conform to the outmoded dictates of the "Four Basic Food Groups," are nevertheless too high in sugar, fat, salt and additives and too deficient in vitamins, minerals and fiber. And many schools have simply abandoned their hot lunch programs, turning the nourishment of their pupils over to vending machine companies which prefer to stock high-profit, long-shelf-life items like candy, soda and snack cakes to fresh fruits and vegetables. A few high schools even operate in-house candy stores to raise money. The teachers in such schools say that the students' behavior is noticeably worse after the candy store opens — but nobody seems to make the connection.

The only way to overcome this sort of influence is to become personally involved. Find out what kind of information is being presented in your child's health and nutrition classes. If you feel the material is unbalanced, make your thoughts known to your child's teacher, to the PTA and to the school board — and be prepared to back up your statements with the sort of research you have read in this book. Organize other nutrition-conscious parents to get non-nourishing products removed from lunch programs and vending machines, and encourage your school to investigate the many ways they can provide food that's both delicious and life-supporting. Don't let them tell you it can't be done — schools all over the nation are doing it right now![5] One courageous fighter for better school lunch programs — Sara Sloan — has developed the Nutra program, a series of classes and workshops for students, teachers and parents, showing them all the value of whole grains and fresh fruits and vegetables. The Nutra program is fun, exciting — and effective.[6]

Do what you can to help your school teach good nutrition. In the meantime ...send a bag lunch. It's not hard — or expensive — to provide your child with a meal that's much more enticing than the garbage the school is offering.

However hard you try to limit the amount of nutritional misinformation your child or teen is exposed to, it's impossible (and probably undesirable) to isolate him or her completely. The ultimate defense is to make sure your children understand why junk food is bad for their bodies and their minds. Let them know they'll have better stamina, they'll feel happier and have more energy to do the things that they want to do if they eat foods that nourish them.

You might also let them know that the proper diet will help them avoid the ravages of acne, give them shinier, more attractive hair, and generally improve the way they look — something any teenager is naturally concerned with.

The nutritional approach also has many positive implications for parents with teens already in trouble. Too many theories have attempted to place the blame for delinquency, neurosis and schizophrenia squarely on the shoulders of the parents. Psychologists and social workers have taken these theories seriously, and have sometimes made families feel extremely guilty for their alleged role in the unbalancing of their child. The result has been to make families uncooperative in the counselor's attempts to help the child — and the process goes nowhere.[7]

Knowing that poor diet, allergies and toxicities can be major contributors to delinquent behavior and mental illness can be a tremendously encouraging thing to parents. It removes much of the senseless mystery imposed by traditional psychiatry, and relieves the anxiety that they have somehow "made the kid crazy." Knowing that mental dysfunction is fundamentally biochemical gives parents great hope that something can be done; moreover, it gives them something to do. They can take a direct part in bringing their child back to full health, rather than simply standing mutely by while the doctor or psychologist takes over.

In short, then, the orthomolecular understanding of the human brain means that parents shape their children's behavior in a way perhaps more profound than teaching them right from wrong. By the way they feed their children, and the way they teach their teens to feed themselves, they help the child develop the sort of healthy nervous system which will help them *discern* right from wrong, and to act in healthy and productive ways. Healthy, happy kids (and adults) simply don't get into trouble. In a sense, parents are the biochemical managers of their children. It is a responsibility they must not neglect, and one they dare not perform in ignorance.

Psychiatry and Psychology

The orthomolecular approach must have every bit as much impact on psychiatrists, psychologists and other types of counselors as it does on parents. But unlike parents, psychiatric professionals tend to be less pragmatic. Rather than exploring whatever works and discarding what does not, professionals must fit studies and techniques into the notions of human behavior they picked up in school. If a therapy or a report makes sense in terms of the latest paradigm of how people think and act, then it is accepted, or at least discussed, no matter whether there's any clinical evidence that it works. If, however, a therapy calls into question the basic models, it is frequently rejected out of hand, regardless of the amount of clinical evidence which supports it.

This is precisely what is now happening in the field of orthomolecular psychiatry. It calls into question all the things psychiatrists, psychologists and doctors have been taught about human behavior. As a result, orthomolecular psychiatry has been reviled in mainstream medical journals, the studies which support it have been simply ignored, the publications which deal with it have been denied listings in important indexes, and the physicians who practice it have been threatened with censure or revocation of their license.[8]

To understand why orthomolecular psychiatry has met such fierce opposition, we need to know a little about the history of psychiatry. Through most of human history, people have been thought of as consisting of two distinct parts: the physical, or body, and the mental, or spirit. This "ghost in the machine" model of the person makes sense in terms of our basic perceptions. We sense our thoughts and emotions directly, while we sense our bodies only secondarily (through sensations of sight, touch, smell, etc.). Thus it seems to make sense that the thing that does the thinking and deciding and wanting (the mind) is a different *sort* of thing than that which does the moving and eating and feeling (the body).

As a result, we make a distinction between "sickness" (when something is wrong with the body itself) and "madness" (when something is wrong with what the body is *doing* — that is, behavior). When we are sick, we seek to cure the body. When we are depressed, frightened, unable to make decisions, or unable to separate reality from hallucination, we try to cure the mind.

But how do we cure the mind? How do we heal the ghost in the machine? Many techniques have been tried through the ages. The earliest notions of mental illness involved demon possession; the rightful ghost was being supplanted by one or more alien, evil ghosts. The solution was thought to involve prayer, or perhaps physical beating. Later it was thought that insanity was a result of some moral defect. The insane person just had a bad ghost inside, and there was nothing to do but lock both it and the machine it inhabited away. This notion led to the establishment of great warehouses for the mentally ill, such as London's notorious Bethlehem Hospital, whose name gives us the modern term "bedlam."

With the advent of Sigmund Freud and his theories in the late 19th and early 20th centuries, psychiatry took a new and, it must be admitted, somewhat more humane turn. Freud divided the mind into the conscious and the unconscious, and postulated that mental illness was caused by internal conflicts generated in childhood. Freud developed psychoanalysis based on his theories, in which the analyst discovered these conflicts by examining the childhood memories of the patient. Once these conflicts were brought to the conscious, the patient could make progress overcoming them, and become sane.

Since Freud there have been many different psychological theories, put forward by eminent researchers like Federn, Jung, Rogers, Meyer, etc. The theories have lead to a plethora of different therapies: dream analysis, family therapy, confrontation therapy, primal scream, client-centered therapy, and hundreds of variations on Freudian psychoanalysis. All are based on the notion that we must cure the ghost in the machine. Even as the science of neurochemistry grew, and researchers learned more and more about how brain chemistry influenced behavior, the psychiatric professions still clung to the notion that the path of mental health lay in dealing with a mind that was somehow disassociated from the body.

While these techniques have been sometimes useful in helping people deal with minor conflicts or "hangups," the fact is that they simply haven't worked in cases of serious mental and behavioral disorders. The evidence is quite clear that traditional psychotherapy has done little or nothing to cure schizophrenia[9] or other psychoses,[10] and that it is ineffective in preventing delinquency[11] or in modifying the behavior of convicted criminals.[12] In fact, psychiatry as it has been practiced has been such a dismal failure that one author has been moved to call it "the impossible profession."[13]

This failure has led many psychiatrists to examine the notion that indeed the mind and the body might not be completely disassociated; that the chemistry and functioning of the brain might have a direct impact on behavior. Two of the founders of the orthomolecular approach, Abram Hoffer and Humphry Osmond, were at the forefront of the biochemical approach in the 1950's as they began their treatment of schizophrenics with massive doses of niacin. Their results were promising, but something happened which forced them into the background of mainstream psychiatry: the invention and marketing of phenothiazines — tranquilizing drugs which immediately dealt with some of the more disturbing symptoms of psychosis.[14]

The orthomolecular approach took a backseat to this new type of chemical intervention for a number of reasons. Psychoactive drugs work within minutes; nutrients and dietary correction take days or weeks to show benefits. Tranquilizers are patentable, and the producers of them stand to make a big profit by advertising them aggressively; vitamins like niacin are inexpensive and easy to get, and so there is little money in publicizing them. There is one other reason that should not be ignored: psychoactive drugs are complex, difficult to synthesize and, of course, very risky; in short, they generate the kind of excitement that turns many doctors on.[15] Vitamins are simple, mundane and harmless — not terribly glamorous.

Yet, for all the commotion generated by the mind drugs, they too are proving to be a psychiatric dead-end. While they deal rapidly with symptoms, they do nothing to cure the disease — that has been left to psychotherapy, which, as we have seen, does little to reverse mental illness. In the meantime, these drugs can be extremely addictive, and can create grotesque side-effects such as tardive dyskinesia (see Chapter Four). Thus, many psychiatrists are coming to realize that this kind of chemical intervention is not much more useful than earlier strategies for coping with mental illness.

As a result, some are returning to the orthomolecular approach. Dr. Jack L. Ward, once a traditional psychotherapist, describes his "conversion" this way:

> ...My practice began to have its frustrating aspects. The heady experiences of being able to communicate with some schizophrenic patients on a highly symbolic or primary level, the identification of "double binds," the demonstration of the workings of the "schizophrenogenic" mother, etc., seemed to have little value in the treatment of my patients. Major tranquilizers and antidepressants were useful, but large doses were necessary and had

> to be continued indefinitely. Too often the dose necessary to control the symptoms also kept the patient on the level of a semi-functioning zombie. And even so, there were relapses. At about this time, I learned from Hoffer and Osmond that massive doses of niacinamide and ascorbic acid could modify the LSD state...[16]

Dr. Allan Cott describes a similar discovery through despair:

> I began an assessment of my discouraging clinical results and faced the appalling reality that after 20 years of general internship, four years of specialty training, and three years of military experience in psychiatry, I had spent the following 22 years treating 25-30 neurotic patients each year! When the use of psychotropics and anti-depressants was introduced, these added a new dimension to the treatment of schizophrenia, but the clinical results, the alarming side effects, and drugging effects patients experienced with the large doses necessary to control their illness, while less discouraging than previous treatments, still led me to continue searching.[17]

Both these men were brought to the orthomolecular approach, and both stayed with it because it worked.

This is perhaps the primary reason why the practice of orthomolecular psychiatry continues to grow, despite the fact that little funding is available for research, and the studies that have been done are largely ignored or suppressed by the mainstream psychiatric media: the approach is extremely successful. Many psychiatrists, frustrated for years at their inability to help the mentally ill with standard treatment methods, are overjoyed at the improvement that megavitamin therapy, dietary correction and allergy prevention can effect. This is how Dr. David Hawkins describes the experience of one agency, the Youth Consultation Service, when they began to experiment with the "medical" (i.e., biochemical) model of mental illness:

> It is expensive and inefficient to try to treat schizophrenia by dealing primarily with the difficult social situations which the patients frequently

> present because of their functional impairment...
>
> When this agency began to experiment with the medical model, they discovered that they could double the effective output of their organization, because the previously unrecognized and undiagnosed illnesses of their clients were now being detected and adequately treated. As the patients clinically improved, the need for extensive social case-work services was greatly reduced.
>
> Following the medical model, we try to correct or compensate for a basic medical defect, and if the treatment method is correct the secondary signs and symptoms will disappear. Normal emotionality will then progressively return, the capacity to form interpersonal relationships will re-emerge, and social functioning will improve...In many patients, therefore, full recovery should occur with no other treatment than strictly medical help.[18]

This success, if it is to be obtained, however, will call for some changes in modern psychiatry. Doctors-in-training will have to be taught the basics of nutrition (something that still doesn't happen in most medical schools[19]) and how diet affects neurochemistry and thus behavior. But more importantly, they will have to abandon the strictly dualistic, "ghost-in-the-machine" image of the human person, and adopt a more wholistic image, an image in which "body" and "mind" are unified aspects of the total individual. This is perhaps the crucial step, and the most difficult; one very respected and highly-placed psychiatrist has adamantly proclaimed, "Even if every other psychiatrist in the country believed in vitamin therapy, I would not believe in it."[20] Fortunately, such irrational rejection of the orthomolecular approach is being overcome; in psychiatric conventions the nutritional and dietary approach is receiving more notice.[21]

The orthomolecular approach is rewarding for the psychiatric *patient* as well as the practitioner. For too long psychiatric patients have been made to feel guilty for their illness. For too long they have been told that their overpowering fears and terrifying sensory distortions were the product of some obscure "search for meaning," were visited upon them by their mothers, or were due to deep internal conflicts over which they had little control. The medical model teaches them that mental illness is a physical disease, like any other, and that it can be treated. Such a revelation is nothing less than the gift of hope, and can greatly increase the cooperation a patient is willing to show in his or her own healing process.[22]

All this is not to say that the orthomolecular approach will make psychotherapy and other types of counseling obsolete. Most of our behavior, and certainly all of our social interactions, are the product both of our biological equipment and our training. The orthomolecular psychiatrist restores the *ability* to live a meaningful and healthy life. As such, metabolic correction is the primary form of treatment. Yet some patients, especially those who have suffered from physical disorders since childhood, will need to learn *how* to interact normally with the environment and the people in it. Thus psychotherapy will still have an important place in the treatment of those with emotional and behavioral disorders.[23]

The Criminal Justice System

In Chapter Four we looked at the inability of the criminal justice system to deal with the enormous workload it faces. Despite the billions of dollars spent annually to secure the blessings of justice, despite the fact that the courts are handling over 3,000 more cases a year now than in 1950,[24] the criminal justice system seems more plagued with problems and inefficiency than ever. The rights of both offenders and victims are being abused daily by a system which, while attempting to be prompt and fair, is in all actuality too overloaded to be either. The result is that justice is perverted almost as frequently as it is upheld.

And what happens after an individual is convicted? The old dream of turning prison houses into modern rehabilitation centers has decayed and crumbled in the light of reality. The fact is that, far from being made more capable of functioning in society, ex-convicts are far more likely to become involved in new crimes after leaving prison. Instead of any sort of rehabilitation, prisoners are subjected to physical deprivation, sexual abuse, official indifference and a refresher course in crime. As a result, the return rate of prison parolees is close to 70 percent. And because the prisons are now crowded far beyond capacity, each new criminal sentenced to incarceration means another criminal who must be released early to make room, sometimes much too soon for any realistic effort at rehabilitation to be made.

All of this inefficiency and waste carries with it a mind-boggling price tag. Nearly $26 billion was spent on the criminal justice system in the United States in 1980, the majority of it on jails and prisons. That's not too hard to believe, when you consider that there are 314,000 inmates serving more than one year in state and federal prisons, and another 158-394 in county and local jails.[25] The story of our criminal justice system is summed up all too simply: wasted money, wasted lives.

Can the orthomolecular approach do anything to alleviate these problems? This is one area where the benefits of treating delinquency and criminality with dietary correction have been convincingly illustrated. My own experience with dietary correction, in which the recidivism rate of my probationers was sharply reduced, is one example, and there are many more. When the Alameda County Probation Department of Oakland, California, cut sugar and sugared foods out of the menu of their juvenile detention centers, they found that their charges became much more manageable, and at the same time there were significant savings in the food budget.[26]

When the San Luis Obispo Juvenile

Probation Department started a Clinical Ecology program, they found a large majority of their probationers had hypoglycemia and other metabolic disorders. Dietary correction was extremely successful in correcting the probationers' behavior problems.[27] Several other American correctional institutions have begun examining the effects of diet on the behavior of their inmates, most with equally encouraging results.

One of the most eloquent cases of the use of the orthomolecular approach in prison reform comes not from the United States, but from Portugal. European prisons are often even worse than American ones. There are, for instance, no separations between hard-core criminals and those convicted of lesser offenses. Crime, drug abuse and the beating of prisoners are common occurrences.

In the midst of this situation, the Unimave Foundation, an organization dedicated to spreading a whole-foods diet to Latin America, has begun instituting its programs in Portuguese prisons, often with impressive results. Prisoners have started demanding that sugar, chemicals and processed foods be removed from their diets, and that they be allowed to have fresh vegetables and whole grains, even if they must buy them with their own pitiful funds and cook them over tiny camp stoves.

When Meg Seaker, managing editor of *East-West Journal,* visited Cadeia Central de Lisboa (Lisbon Central Prison) in March of 1982, she saw some inspiring things: hardened criminals who had gained tranquility and self-confidence for the first time in their lives. Some of the worst prisoners in Portugal were now reporting a spiritual intensity to their lives — a far cry from the hopelessness instilled by the American prison system![28]

If such programs could be instituted in the prisons and jails of the United States, it would undoubtedly go a long way toward enabling the criminal justice system to do the job it is supposed to do. If the incredibly high recidivism rate could be improved by even as much as 50 percent (and some trials of the orthomolecular approach suggest this is possible[29]), thousands of cases could be removed from the dockets of the criminal courts each year. This would not only make time and free resources so that more people could get swift and fair treatment, it would help end the situation in which convicts must be prematurely released to make room for others.

It would, in addition, make it possible for criminals to be sent somewhere where they could receive real, positive rehabilitation. Our prisons and detention centers could become something more than warehouses for the socially outcast. The savings in money, time and resources now wasted on caging human beings would be substantial, and the possibility of transforming dangerous wards of the state into productive citizens would be priceless.

Society As A Whole

We have looked at some specific areas in which a realization of the orthomolecular approach could have an enormous positive impact. But we ought to remember that diet influences the behavior of *everyone,* not just juvenile delinquents, mental patients and prisoners. Hypoglycemia may affect literally millions of Americans,[30] and malnutrition may afflict a large percentage of the nation's population.[31] Who can begin to estimate what this means in terms of the loss of human potential? One study has suggested that low blood sugar may actually have taken a direct and violent toll on human life, by contributing to the increase in accidental death.[32] How many lives are ruined by unrecognized alcoholism, depression, inability to learn, and sensory distortion? We have seen that all these emotional and behavioral problems have their metabolic roots, and that all can be influenced by diet.

If the orthomolecular concept could be accepted throughout society, the possible benefits would be beyond estimate. I do not want to suggest that turning the world on to a whole foods diet would immediately bring the end of all human problems. But when you consider the possibility of living in a safer, saner, more productive world, a world where the tragedies of human sickness and mental illness could be radically reduced, you don't have to be a utopian dreamer to yearn to make this kind of world a reality.

It is hard to say how such a drastic change in the eating habits of the Western world could come about, especially when one considers how entrenched the huge processed food conglomerates are in our economy.[33] One must remember, as well, that the kind of nutritional decimation which processed foods undergo was devised in order to minimize costs of production and maximize profits. Thus our junk food diet has been inspired by free enterprise, and it's a little difficult to see how the people who control our food supply could be made to change their ways short of some massive direct government action. Does this mean, then, that there is no hope?

I don't believe so. Let me direct these concluding comments specifically to parents. I don't know of a single parent who wouldn't do all he or she could to make their children healthy and happy or give them a better world to grow up in. Changing the world is something beyond what can be expected of any parent; but feeding your children the proper foods, giving their bodies and their minds the nutrients they require, is the very least that any parent would want to do.

This is the beautiful part, the reason why I have so much hope. If enough parents are concerned enough about nutrition to give their kids a natural, whole foods diet, many kids will grow stronger in body and mind. It seems obvious, in light of the material I have presented in this book, that an increase in well-nourished kids will bring about a decrease in delinquency, criminality, learning disabilities, aggressiveness and a host of other behavioral problems. In short, the world would become a better, safer, saner place. So by feeding your children responsibly, encouraging exercise, and spreading the word about the link between diet, health and behavior, you can actually do more about changing the world than all the politicians, philosphers or soldiers who have ever lived. This, I believe, is our greatest hope for the future.

NOTES

[1]Lendon Smith, *Feed Your Kids Right,* (New York: Dell Publishing Company, Inc., 1979), p. 228.

[2]Helen G. First, "Anatomy of Resistance to the Emergent Paradigm: Orthomolecular Medicine," *Journal of Orthomolecular Psychiatry,* 1980, Vol. 9 No. 4, pp. 253-262.

[3]A. Hoffer, "Behavioral Nutrition," *Journal of Orthomolecular Psychiatry,* 1979, Vol. 8 No. 3, pp. 169-175.

[4]Greg Moyer, "School Daze," *Nutrition Action,* September 1982, pp. 6-9.

[5]Scott Knickelbine, *Diet and Alcoholism,* Nutritional Resource Center (P.O. Box 2107, Manitowoc, Wisconsin 54220).

[6]Sara Sloan, *From Classroom to Cafeteria,* (Food Service

Program, Fulton County Schools, 786 Cleveland Avenue, S.W., Atlanta, Georgia 30315.)

[7]Cynthia C. Bisbee, "Patient Education in Psychiatric Illness," *Journal of Orthomolecular Psychiatry,* 1979, Vol. 8 No. 4, pp. 239-247.

[8]First, "Anatomy of Resistance," op. cit.

[9]Humphry Osmond, "The Background to the Niacin Treatment," in David Hawkins and Linus Pauling, ed.s, *Orthomolecular Psychiatry,* (San Francisco: W.H. Freeman and Company, 1973), pp. 194-201.

[10]J. Kinross-Wright, article, *Journal of the American Medical Association,* 1967, No. 200, pp. 461-464.

[11]Joan McCord, "A Thirty-Year Follow-up of Treatment Effects," *The American Psychologist,* March 1978, pp. 284-289.

[12]A. Hoffer, "Crime, Punishment and Treatment," *Journal of Orthomolecular Psychiatry,* 1979, Vol. 8 No. 3, pp. 193-199.

[13]*The Impossible Profession,* (New York: Viking, 1981).

[14]Osmond, "The Background to the Niacin Treatment," op. cit.

[15]First, "Anatomy of Resistance," op. cit.

[16]Jack L. Ward, "Conversion to Orthomolecular Treatment," *Journal of Orthomolecular Psychiatry,* 1977, Vol. 2 No. 2, pp. 183-185.

[17]Allan Cott, "From The Traditional Approach to Biochemical Treatment," *Journal of Orthomolecular Psychiatry,* 1977, Vol. 2 No. 2, pp. 178-182.

[18]David Hawkins, "The Orthomolecular Approach to Diagnosis of Schizophrenia," in Hawkins and Pauling, *Orthomolecular Psychiatry,* p. 601.

[19]First, "Anatomy of Resistance," op. cit.

[20]Ibid.

[21]William H. Philpott, "Observation of the 1978 American Psychiatric Convention," *Journal of Orthomolecular Psychiatry,* 1979, Vol. 8 No. 4, pp. 273-274.

[22]Bisbee, "Patient Education," op. cit.

[23]Ibid.

[24]*1981 Statistical Abstract of the United States,* (Washington, D.C.: U.S. Department of Commerce Bureau of the Census, 1989), p. 184.

[25]*Statistical Abstract,* p. 184.

[26]Alexander Schauss, *Diet, Crime and Delinquency,* (Berkeley, California: Parker House, 1981), pp. 11-13.

[27]Ibid.

[28]Meg Seaker, "Fighting Crime with Diet: A Report from Portugal," *East-West Journal,* July 1982, pp. 26-34.

[29]Alexander Schauss, "Differential Outcomes among Probationers Comparing Orthomolecular Approaches to Conventional Casework/Counseling," *Journal of Orthomolecular Psychiatry,* 1979, Vol. 8 No. 3, pp. 158-168.

[30]Marilyn Light, Executive Director of the Adrenal Metabolic Research Society of the Hypoglycemic Foundation, as cited in William Dufty, *Sugar Blues,* (New York: Warner Books, 1976), p. 21.

[31]Carl C. Pfeiffer, *Mental and Elemental Nutrients,* (New Canaan, Connecticut: Keats Publishing, Inc., 1975), p. 3.

[32]Broda O. and Charlotte W. Barnes, *Hope for Hypoglycemia,* (Fort Collins, Colorado: Robinson Press, 1978), pp. 41-49.

[33]Louis Junker, *Nutrition and Economy: Some Observa-*

[33]Louis Junker, *Nutrition and Economy: Some Observations on Diet and Disease in the American Food Power System,* unpublished paper delivered at the Western Social Science Association Meetings — Association for Institutional Thought, April 1981.

APPENDIX

Suggested Reading

Aerobics by Kenneth H. Cooper, M.D., M.P.H. (Bantam Books).

Allergies and Your Child by Doris J. Rapp, M.D. (Holt, Rinehart and Winston).

An Alternative Approach to Allergies by Theron G. Randolph, M.D. and Ralph W. Moss, Ph.D. (Lippincott & Crowell, Publishers).

Biochemical Individuality by Roger J. Williams, Ph.D. (University of Texas Press).

Body, Mind and Sugar by E.M. Abrahamson, M.D. and A.W. Pezet (Avon Books).

Brain Allergies by William H. Philpott, M.D. and Dwight K. Kalita, Ph.D. (Keats Publishing, Inc.).

Brand Name Guide to Sugar by Ira L. Shannon, D.M.D., M.S.D. (Nelson-Hall Books).

Diet, Crime and Delinquency by Alexander Schauss (Parker House Books).

Dr. Mandell's 5-Day Allergy Relief System by Marshall Mandell, M.D. and L. Scanlon (Thomas Y. Crowell Publisher).

Earl Mindell's Vitamin Bible by Earl Mindell (Rawson, Wade Publishers).

Feed Your Kids Right by Lendon Smith, M.D. (Delta Books).

Fighting the Food Giants by Paul Stitt, M.S., with Mark Knickelbine and Scott Knickelbine (Natural Press).

Look Younger, Live Longer by Gayelord Hauser (Fawcett Crest Books).

Mental and Elemental Nutrients by Carl C. Pfeiffer, Ph.D., M.D. (Keats Publishing, Inc.).

Nutrition Against Disease, by Roger J. Williams, Ph.D. (Bantam Books).

Orthomolecular Nutrition by Abram Hoffer, Ph.D., M.D. and Morton Walker, D.P.M. (Keats Publishing, Inc.).

Orthomolecular Psychiatry, Linus Pauling, Ph.D. and David Hawkins, M.D. editors (W.H. Freeman and Company).

A Physician's Handbook on Orthomolecular Medicine, Roger J. Williams, Ph.D. and Dwight K. Kalita, Ph.D. editors (Pergamon Press).

Psychodietetics by E. Cheraskin, M.D., D.M.D. and W.M. Ringsdorf, Jr., D.M.D., M.S., with Arline Brecher (Bantam Books).

Sugar Blues by William Dufty (Warner Books).

The Supernutrition Handbook by Patrick Mooney (self-published; available through Natural Press).

Tracking Down Hidden Food Allergies by William Crook, M.D. (Professional Books).

ORGANIZATIONS TO CONTACT

Huxley Institute, 219 East 31st Street, New York, NY 10016. Director: Albrecht Heyer, Phone: 212/683-9455.

Canadian Schizophrenia Foundation, 2229 Broad Street, Regina, Saskatchewan, S4P 1Y7.

Nutritional Resource Center, 104 N. 8th Street, P.O. Box 2107, Manitowoc, WI 54220. Contact: Ms. Ellen Bonnin, Phone: 414/682-0738.

International Graphoanalysis Society, Inc., Dept. 29337, 111 North Canal Street, Chicago, IL 60606. Director: Harold L. Wise, Ph.D.

WANT TO LEARN MORE ABOUT DIET AND BEHAVIOR?

THE EXPERTS ACCLAIM BARBARA REED

"At last! Here in Barbara Reed's own words is the story of her celebrated discovery of the strong links between criminality and diet. Her story is a fascinating one..."

— Bernard Rimland, Ph.D.,
Director,
Institute for Child
Behavior Research

"Barbara Reed has provided invaluable information on the links between diet and behavior to myself and the entire profession."

— Lendon Smith, M.D.
Author,
Feed Your Kids Right

"This volume is an eye-opener for those professionally involved in law enforcement."

— Marshall Mandel, M.D.
Author,
Dr. Mandel's 5-day
Allergy Relief System

"I was amazed at the dramatic results in persons who were placed on probation to her through my court."

— Judge William B. Pike
Municipal Court of
Cuyahoga Falls, Ohio

"I have read *Food, Teens and Behavior* — in fact, I could not put it down. I cannot speak strongly enough, nor can I say too strongly to parents, health professionals or those in other helping professions — Read this book!"

**— Mary L. Friedel, Director
Guardian Angel Home,
Joliet, Illinois**

"Barbara Reed is one of the pioneers in studying the relationship of malnutrition to crime and in bringing this to the attention of the medical and scientific world."

**— A. Hoffer, M.D., Ph.D.
Editor-in-Chief,**
Journal of Orthomolecular Psychiatry

"Our staff is sold that there's a tie-up among diet, emotions and behavior. The Barbara Reed approach has not only helped clients, but several staff members, to live healthier, more effective lives."

**— Robert E. Golden
Former New York State
Probation Commissioner**

"I have seen the positive results of Barbara's dietary program and I'm very pleased with the low rearrest rate. I'm a wholehearted supporter of her program!"

**— Judge James M. Bierce
Municipal Court of
Cuyahoga Falls, Ohio**